The Uncomfortable Truth

Anna Mathur is a psychotherapist and bestselling author. She's passionate about taking therapy out of the consulting room: sharing her personal and professional experiences online. She offers supportive insights on Instagram (@annamathur), via online courses and in-person events, and through her incredibly popular podcast, *The Therapy Edit*. Anna's podcast has now released over 250 episodes and received over three million downloads, with guests including Fearne Cotton, Sophie Ellis-Bextor, Anna Whitehouse, Holly Tucker, Giovanna Fletcher and Liz Earle.

The Uncomfortable Truth

Change Your Life by Taming 10 of
Your Mind's Greatest Fears

Anna Mathur

PENGUIN LIFE

AN IMPRINT OF

PENGUIN BOOKS

PENGUIN LIFE

UK | USA | Canada | Ireland | Australia
India | New Zealand | South Africa

Penguin Life is part of the Penguin Random House group of companies
whose addresses can be found at global.penguinrandomhouse.com.

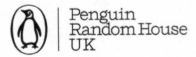

First published 2024
003

Copyright © Anna Mathur, 2024

Set in 12/18pt TT Commons Classic
Typeset by Jouve (UK), Milton Keynes
Printed and bound in Great Britain by Clays Ltd, Elcograf S.p.A.

The authorized representative in the EEA is Penguin Random House Ireland,
Morrison Chambers, 32 Nassau Street, Dublin D02 YH68

A CIP catalogue record for this book is available from the British Library

ISBN: 978-0-241-70719-7

www.greenpenguin.co.uk

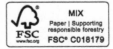

MIX
Paper | Supporting
responsible forestry
FSC® C018179

Penguin Random House is committed to a
sustainable future for our business, our readers
and our planet. This book is made from Forest
Stewardship Council® certified paper.

Dear Reader,

I dedicate this book to you. Because you deserve far more than to spend your whole life living a half-life.

'One thing I feel clear about is that it's important not to let your life live you. Otherwise, you end up at forty feeling like you haven't really lived. What have I learned? Perhaps to live now, so that at fifty I won't look back upon my forties with regret'

– Irvin D. Yalom, *When Nietzsche Wept*

Contents

Welcome

Our fear of bad things happening has our mind telling terrifying stories that steal our focus away from the good things happening right in front of us. We worry about being disliked, so much so that we lose chunks of ourselves pleasing others. We go so far trying to avoid the truth of our inevitable death that we prevent ourselves from truly embracing the life that we have.

What if the real answer to living a happier life isn't avoiding the inevitable, uncomfortable truths, as many of us spend our time doing, but instead choosing to stare them square in the face?

From a young age, I have had to face one of those uncomfortable truths of life head-on.

I am going to die.

I was eight when my younger sister was diagnosed with a terminal brain tumour in her tiny four-year-old head. Lives that had revolved around school, seeing grandparents and playing in the surrounding woodland were now filled with hospital corridors, sickness and scans. We lived in the painful limbo land that fell between a diagnosis and death. We found joy in the waiting, don't get me wrong, but life was a dance between moments of acknowledgement and denial, acceptance and avoidance.

I remember lying in bed thinking that if my sister died, I'd simply have to die too. I didn't believe that it would be possible to live with a broken heart. Life felt too risky, love felt too vulnerable. It would be better simply not to live or to love. My eight-year-old mind also recognized the heartbreak my parents felt. Would I want them to be sad about my death too? Absolutely not. So instead of seeking death, I did everything in my power to avoid any more loss. Theirs and mine. I spent years fearing my own cancer or the sickness of anyone I loved. Health anxiety stole my sleep and my peace as my mind skipped to the worst-case scenario every time someone complained of a headache. The news of the death of someone I didn't even know would replay through my head like a backing track.

At school I faced another uncomfortable truth: that some people wouldn't accept me regardless of how well behaved or well intentioned I was. I had a teacher who bullied me. To this day, I still don't know why. I do know, however, that in each year group she taught, there was one child who'd face the confusing discomfort of her disapproval. I did everything I could to appease her, assuming that if she disliked me, there must be a reason, and the reason lay with me. I'm sure this experience was part of the reason I spent the next almost thirty years of my life in the relentless, exhausting pursuit of acceptance. Acceptance from everyone.

A little later in life, aged twenty-three, I began my postgraduate studies to become a psychotherapist at Regent's University London. We studied different approaches to therapy, including a focus on the 'existential' approach, which acknowledges that many of our anxieties and insecurities come down to how we relate to and accept life's fundamental certainties and uncertainties.

I quickly fell in love with the work of Irvin D. Yalom. Yalom certainly wasn't the first theorist to share this existential way of making sense of life. Philosophers Nietzsche, Kierkegaard, Heidegger and Sartre all explored concepts around our personal responsibility in finding meaning. And

May and Tillich were known for bringing this form of philosophy into the mainstream through their work.

However, I found Yalom's take on existentialism particularly warm and hopeful. In his book *Existential Psychotherapy* he suggested that, as humans, we grapple with these four main themes, which are the inescapable 'givens' of life:

- **Death** Death is an inevitable and inescapable part of life.
- **Freedom** We have the freedom to make choices that impact our lives.
- **Isolation** We have connection with others, yet we exist as single beings in the world.
- **Meaninglessness** We seek meaning but we don't have inherent meaning in this world.

Yalom, along with other existential thinkers, suggested that how we understand these 'givens' can determine whether we feel heightened anxiety and fear, or alternatively, a sense of compassion and acceptance as we navigate life.

As a therapist who incorporates existentialism into my practice, I aim to work with my clients to help them become more accepting of life's certainties: that death comes to us all and there is much outside the realm of our control.

At first, as a student, I found the existentialist module deeply depressing. I didn't want to think about death; I wanted to avoid thinking about bad things happening. Considering my freedom to make both good and damaging life choices forced me to confront the responsibility, power and vulnerability I had in shaping my life. I tussled with the fourth given, that of 'meaninglessness', as personally I drew meaning from my belief in a higher power. Yet I also acknowledged that many of the anxieties I experienced were around the very truths we were encouraging our clients to come to terms with.

I began to understand how existential therapy is all about finding a balance between being aware and accepting of these givens of life, while not being overwhelmed by anxiety at their inevitability.

My work is about encouraging my clients to find their own meaning and purpose, as life won't present it to them. It's about supporting them as they face their vulnerability, or the enormity of the responsibility they have in making decisions, while accepting that life's losses and curve balls will inevitably come along and nudge or reroute their path.

I empower my clients to find their potential, while also acknowledging their mortality. I seek to hold space for them as they contend with their anxiety, while encouraging them to move forward with living more intentionally. We all exist with this internal conflict, trying to live with intention, while being aware (consciously or subconsciously) that ultimately we lack control over the outcome.

For years I worked with clients to help them address the anxiety of the unknown, but it would take a long time for me to recognize that the best way to live fully is to seek acceptance of the unknown itself. We can exhaust ourselves trying to avoid the elephant in the room, contorting our lives around it or defending ourselves against it through busyness or numbing behaviours like alcohol, social media or consuming. Or we can look it square in the face and say, 'Hey. You're here for good, so let's find a way to live together.'

The truth is that all the difficult stuff in my life – the anxiety, the need to numb my reality, the people-pleasing,

the perfectionism – all of these things arose from my
desperate attempt to avoid the uncomfortable truths
being, well, true. Yet in accepting the uncomfortable
truths, my life has actually become far more intentional
and fulfilling, and less uncomfortable!

I used to be a 'yes' woman through and through. Ask me
to do something and you'd have a 'yes' before you'd
paused for breath. Saying 'yes' was my currency. I
believed that spending all my time and energy fulfilling
the desires and needs of others was what made me
acceptable. However, as the years went by, I struggled
with hidden burnout and resentment. As I began to realize
how much each 'yes' was costing me, I started placing
boundaries and saying 'no' more often. Sure, it hasn't
been easy, and some difficult conversations have been
had, but now my yeses are far more authentic, my
relationships more two-sided and my behind-the-scenes
less burnt-out.

My life has been changed by choosing to befriend the
elephant in the room. And this book is an invitation for you
to join me.

Introduction

In his book *If Only It Were True* Marc Levy challenges us with this scenario. Imagine your bank account was credited with $86,400 each morning. So far, so very good, right? The catch is that at the end of each day the balance is wiped and nothing can be carried over. Your mind is likely buzzing with ways you'd try to withdraw and use every last cent so that it didn't go to waste. He says that, in the same way, every day we are gifted 86,400 seconds that we cannot keep, save or carry over. 'You must live in the present on today's deposits. Invest it so as to get from it the utmost in health, happiness and success! The clock is running. Make the most of it.'

I wonder what feelings you are left with on reading that scenario. Panic, regret, guilt, empowerment? For me it feels like empowerment, but it also feels like pressure. Pressure to make the most of every second. It feels like grief. Grief that I've not squeezed every one of my 86,400 seconds for health, happiness and success. This challenge fuels anxiety, that I'm not living as I should, that my mind and attention are scattered, and I often lack the calmness and patience I need in order to be present.

Regardless of how you felt as you considered what you'd do with that eye-watering daily figure of cash, or the sobering figure of seconds, this book is all about finding hope. It's about finding acceptance of the fact that life is limited, while embracing realistic ways to live a full, messy, very human, fulfilling life.

If you feel anxiety bubbling as you turn your focus to these big themes, rest assured. This book eases anxiety, but not with tools and tips for breathing exercises and reframing thoughts (although you'll find some of these woven throughout which you may benefit from). This book will teach you to calm your anxiety not by sidestepping the symptoms but by taking a long, hard look at your deepest fears.

If we distilled anxiety down over a Bunsen burner, the racing heart, pacing mind, sweaty palms, broken sleep and churning stomach would all evaporate. We'd look down into the beaker to view the molten remnants and we'd find these ten uncomfortable truths.

We spend millions of pounds and hours numbing our fears. The alcohol industry is roaring. In much-needed moments of nothingness, we reach for our phones to scroll lest our emotions and anxieties dominate rare stillness. We pipe sounds into our ears so that we don't have to think. We spend our lives finding new ways to skirt around the truths of life, and the more we avoid them, the more we affirm that they are something to be avoided at all cost.

But avoidance of life's truths carries the highest price of all. We see burnout, perfectionism, addiction, anxiety, people-pleasing, grief and so, so much shame.

Through the course of this book you'll come to realize that many of the challenges you experience in life can be attributed to avoidance of one or more of these ten truths. And as you move into a place of radical acceptance, you'll find yourself living more freely and intentionally, with more presence and confidence than ever before.

I've spent a lot of my life trying to ensure that good things happen, that everyone likes me and that I do not fail. I've devoted copious headspace to ruminating over the times I've done bad things, accidentally or on purpose. I've exhausted myself in the relentless pursuit of doing everything well, and beaten myself up for not being fully present in my life. I have lost sleep as my mind has played out painful images of those I love getting sick.

I was fed up with my constant attempts to control the outcomes of the uncontrollable. I'd become a master at speculating. I'd lived on the hamster wheel of pursuing perfection, failing and trying again. Was this life, I wondered? The constant dodging and avoidance of failure and death? The constant undertone of worry and anxiety? The constant ache of not-good-enoughness?

One same-old day I decided I'd do things differently.

'Some people don't like me. I am going to fail. I am going to die,' I muttered under my breath. These three truths underpinned my nightmares and my deepest fears. All my life, I'd spent so much of myself trying to secure likeability and success, and fearing death.

What if I faced the truth head-on, instead of spending my time running from it?

As I muttered these three foreboding sentences under my breath, something incredible began to happen. Instead of feeling more fear, I felt freer. Instead of exhaustion, I felt a fresh lightness.

I took out my phone and started to list other truths that I'd spent too much time trying to avoid. 'I'll never find balance,' I typed. 'I am not good enough. Bad things will happen. I can't always be fully present.' As I wrote these fundamental truths, I didn't feel defeated, but empowered.

I realized that we try so hard to control the things that we cannot control in pursuit of a contented life, but we aren't content at all, really. Are we? We're all a little sad, scared and tired.

In facing the uncomfortable truths of life head-on, we can receive the invitation to live more authentically, more fully.

In recognizing the truth that not everyone will like us, we can stop feeling so deeply pained when we displease someone. In admitting that we simply cannot be consistently present and focused on the moment in front of us, we can relieve ourselves of pressure and guilt, and focus on slowing down where we can. Instead of lying awake fearful of death, we can make decisions with confident intentionality, because life is short and we deserve to live it fully.

There is always a cost to avoiding the truth, because these fundamental truths don't change. It becomes more and more exhausting to dance around them. I have spoken to so many people in their sixties and seventies who profess that caring less about being liked by everyone has been a wonderful gift that has come with age. 'I wish I could tell my younger self not to care,' they say. Well, my hope is that we begin learning to accept these truths long before the perspective of age or burnout forces us to.

So, as you move through ten of the uncomfortable truths of life, you will find that in accepting them they actually make life more beautiful. You'll discover that in running from life's truths, in an attempt to live an authentic and fulfilled life, you've actually been denying yourself the very same thing.

We are going to learn to embrace all that we've spent years trying to escape. We are going to try a different way.

How to read this book

I encourage you to read this book slowly. Let the truth of each chapter settle before you move to the next. Not every truth will feel like one you need to accept, either because you already have an acceptance of that uncomfortable truth, or because you feel too anxious and defensive against it.

If the uncomfortable truth doesn't feel like one that you'd benefit from addressing, then you can of course move past it. However, I'd encourage you to read it anyway as you never know what conversations might arise, or how pondering a truth that you already have deep acceptance of might serve you in an unexpected way. There will be some chapters that feel too big to turn to, but I promise you we will take it gently.

As a psychotherapist, I have spent hundreds of hours sitting with people who have experienced trauma in the light of these truths. You will benefit from many client anecdotes and stories throughout this book. Please be assured that names and details have been amended beyond all recognition, and where likeness is evident, full permission has been obtained.

So while I have sat with many clients as they've grappled with these themes, I am also someone who has spent most of my own life doing everything within my power to avoid these truths (yet also lying awake for hours in anxious contemplation of them). I know that, for some, skimming the contents list alone will raise the heart rate. But by the end of the book you'll feel very differently.

In each chapter, we will gently approach one of the ten uncomfortable truths. We will reflect on what it costs us to avoid facing the uncomfortable truth. We will reflect on why we feel driven to deny that truth. Finally, we'll consider what we can gain from embracing it instead, and I'll share five tangible ways to live with the truth.

You will find a mantra in every chapter, a simple line to ruminate over as you focus on each truth, along with three journal points to guide you in delving deeper into self-reflection should you find them helpful.

Make this book yours. Underline parts of it, turn down corners of chapters and pages you need to revisit, and scribble your thoughts into the margins. The more you take ownership of the words within this book, the more power and freedom you will claim.

1.

Some People Don't Like Me

Diving headfirst into the uncomfortable truth

People don't like you. There, I said it. People don't like me either. Not 'people as a whole', just some people. You will be walking around, standing in queues, doing your best, and someone will have decided they don't like you. Some people won't like you for reasons they can explain – maybe it's something you've done or not done. Perhaps they can't even put their finger on quite why they don't like you, but they don't all the same.

People who don't even know you have decided they don't like you. Someone sitting in the car behind you has sworn at you, while someone at your workplace has gone

1

home and complained about you. You have had many feelings come your way, whether you've been aware of it or not: dislike, judgement, assumption, even hatred. There are subsections of society who will have already chosen to dislike you because of how you look or where you were born, neither of which you can do anything about.

There are some people who don't like you, and it has absolutely nothing whatsoever to do with you at all. Nothing you could do would change that, no act of kindness, no pleading, pleasing or torrent of self-explanation.

How does it feel to read those words in black and white? Breathe them in and absorb them. Notice how they sit in your body and what thoughts come to mind. Perhaps many of those words already swirl through your mind on a tide of anxiety and rumination. Maybe you feel a swell of discomfort arise as you read everything you try to avoid thinking about.

'I parked my car at the supermarket and went in to do my shopping,' my client Tamsin shared with me one session. 'I came back to find that I couldn't open my boot because someone had parked their car right up against it, end to end. When the owner returned to his car I expected him to be apologetic, but instead he was aggressive and ranted at me for having such a sizeable car. "I'm sick of people like you and your big cars thinking you own the place," he shouted. My heart was racing. I wanted to cry. I tried to justify myself. "I have three teenagers and a dog!" I said. However, it was clear he didn't care. It was also clear that him parking against my car wasn't an accident.'

My client found herself in a situation in which someone disliked her based on his own preconceived ideas and judgements. She described feeling enraged at his behaviour and at the same time 'feeling like a kid being told off for something I hadn't done wrong'. We considered how this man's dislike of her had little to do with who she was as an individual, and affirmed how she wasn't doing anything 'wrong' in parking her car in a supermarket car park.

The truth that someone will dislike you is often woven through with anxious thoughts. In this chapter, I am going to help remove that heart-pace-increasing, sleep-stealing element of anxiety and, in place, guide you to welcome fresh acceptance.

My story

A few years ago, I was sitting at traffic lights, picking some peanut butter off my jeans. Out of the corner of my eye, I saw some movement in my rear-view mirror and glanced up to see what the person behind me was flapping about. They looked furious. It didn't take me long to realize that they were miming a mobile phone and gesticulating 'no' at me. I wasn't on my phone. I was picking peanut butter off my jeans.

Regardless of what I was or wasn't doing, my heart rate rocketed. I related to Tamsin in feeling somehow threatened. Suddenly I was eight years old, being told off by an angry teacher. The lights changed to green and I was forced to drive off before I had a chance to respond with my own charade of explanation. I felt her anger move through my body like shock waves. Her furrowed face lurched into my consciousness, followed by a deep uneasiness. I later told a friend, who laughed and said she'd have responded in a very different way. 'I'd have told her with my eyes where to go,' she shared. This intrigued me, shining a light on how much my concern with what other people thought about me, even a stranger in traffic, had so much power over how I felt.

The woman in the car behind me didn't like me. Whether it was momentary or whether it was fuelled by a recent experience she'd had of dangerous driving due to mobile phone usage, I'll never know. But it is just a small tale in the library of examples I have of being impacted by people not liking me, whether true or perceived, whether justified or through misunderstanding. I have other stories in which I've contorted my personality, lied, steamrollered my own boundaries, and confused myself and others in my attempts to ensure people like me. Because for me, for much of my life, not being liked has been my fear, my pain and my driver to do better.

But that changed. I realized that the way to more meaningful relationships and healthier self-esteem isn't to ensure that as many people like me as much as possible, but instead to grow in acceptance that some people simply don't, won't and can't. American philosopher Elbert Hubbard wrote in his book *Little Journeys to the Homes of American Statesmen* that, 'If you would escape moral and physical assassination, do nothing, say nothing, be nothing.' Now, we cannot live our lives doing, saying and being nothing. And would we want to live so small that we slipped under everyone's radar, never shocked anyone, never moved anyone, never challenged anything, never shared enough of ourselves to make a wave in someone's life or the world itself? If we want to live more fully, we must come to terms with the truth that our lives will be disturbing somehow. Like a teaspoon stirring a cup of tea. If you want good tea, you have to move the spoon. If we want a good life, we have to be willing to create waves and ripples around us.

So, now, gesticulate at me in traffic and perhaps my heart will skip a beat because old habits die hard. Then I'll either nod with acknowledgement if I think it's well placed, or find my breath in the acceptance that I will be misunderstood and disliked sometimes, and that's part of existing as a human amidst others. We will explore the uncomfortable truth of being misunderstood more in Chapter 7.

Why deny?

Why do we feel the need to work so hard to try to get others to like us? Why is the truth that some people won't so hard to stomach? Why does it prompt such anxiety and shame for so many of us?

Above all, we humans are innately pack animals. We need to be accepted in order to be protected. The feeling that may rise up within us when we don't feel accepted is a reaction to this. In my session with Tamsin, we gave voice to that part of her which felt threatened as the fellow shopper shouted at her in the car park. We acknowledged how we have a deep human need to be accepted and understood. Being liked by others means we're more likely to thrive and be supported in our community. If you think about the people in your life who you really like, the chances are that you'll also feel an element of care and protectiveness towards them. You want them to be okay, they matter to you. If they're having a tough time, you might seek ways to help them.

Throw your mind back to school years. That yearning to be a part of a group or a clique isn't just culturally encouraged, it speaks of a deep human desire to belong. The problem is that the need to belong in order to feel safe can progress into a need to be accepted by everyone we come across, even those we don't actually know.

If this truth is one you struggle with, then it will be helpful to understand why. I find that understanding why we find it hard to accept the truth enables us to move from a place of self-criticism to self-compassion. Prior to understanding why, for most of my life, I needed people to like me, I'd feel frustrated at myself. Why can't I say 'no'? Why do I lack confidence around certain people? Why do I end up doing things half-heartedly because I am full of resentment for agreeing to do it in the first place?

Wanting to be liked by others and *needing* to be liked are two quite different things. Wanting to be liked drives us to be considerate and respectful. It ensures we think about others and consider how our words and actions might impact them. Caring about being liked means we'll seek to respond to others with compassion and empathy, and our relationships are often all the richer for it.

Needing to be liked, on the other hand, is very different. It has undertones of fear and sometimes even desperation. We need to be liked because we need more than just the inner smile that comes when someone is appreciative of us; we need it because our self-esteem and sense of worthiness depend on it. Perhaps we need it because we've lacked the anchoring sense of being accepted, warts and all, by the few people in our lives who truly had the power to tell us and teach us how deserving of love we were.

The more clarity I gained as to why I feared being disliked by or displeasing others, the more compassion I had towards myself. Compassion doesn't say: 'Oh well, this is why I am the way I am.' Compassion isn't defeatist, that's victimhood. Compassion can be highly mobilizing. It says: 'Here's the explanation, now what can we do to free you up somehow?'

In the case of my client Tamsin, she identified that in childhood she often felt left out by her much older siblings. 'They'd make fun of the games I wanted to play, so I felt lonely and excluded. I did everything I could to try and prove that I could be grown up, like them. All I ever wanted was to feel accepted by them.' Thus feeling disliked by the man in the car park touched on this deeper meaning of what being liked meant to her.

Here are some reasons you might be denying the truth that some people don't like you.

- **You don't like yourself** Do you like yourself? Do you believe that you are deserving of kindness? If you struggle with low self-esteem and feel inherently flawed and unlikeable, then you can experience an insatiable need to please others in order to feel deserving of relationships. Realizing you're not liked can act as confirmation of your deepest narrative, that you aren't likeable. But, trust me, the whole world singing your praises won't be enough to convince you otherwise if you don't like yourself.

- **You don't experience enough deep acceptance from others** Consider someone in your life who deeply knows and accepts you, despite your flaws, toxic traits and weaknesses. Then consider someone who doesn't know you well at all. Now, who of those two people truly gets to say whether you're likeable or not? The more accepted we feel by those who know us best, the less uncomfortable is the truth that not everyone will like us.

- **You've been taught that you aren't likeable** When we are young, we rely on others to keep us safe and show us that we have value. If you have grown up being mistreated or misinformed, then at some point you will have felt unsafe physically, emotionally or otherwise. Being seen as 'bad' or unliked can end up being equated to feeling unsafe, rather than simply a truth we have to accept. Knowing others like you, regardless of the cost, feels safer.

- **Only part of you has been treated as acceptable** Perhaps you have experienced a time in which an element of your character or body has been repeatedly criticized. Perhaps you were taught that only certain, pleasing emotions were acceptable, so you had to suppress or reject parts of yourself in order to feel acceptable to caregivers. Again, in this situation, feeling liked by others works to meet the deep human need for acceptance and belonging.

- **Rejection has been traumatic** If you have experienced a traumatic rejection, you may have felt alone or uncared for. Perhaps someone else's difficulty in accepting others meant that you've felt 'wrong' or 'unlikeable'. Being disliked is a mini rejection and can trigger feelings of shame and even physical pain. Ensuring others like you is, therefore, a mode of self-protection.

I hope these words have stirred compassion towards yourself, where there may have been frustration and criticism. With that in mind, let's look at the benefits of accepting the truth that not everyone will like you.

The benefits of embracing this uncomfortable truth

Knowing the benefits of embracing this uncomfortable truth of life is so empowering. Here are some of the benefits you can enjoy as you choose to start walking a different path.

- **More confidence in the decisions you make** When you worry about what others think, the decisions you make are often tainted by a fear of how people will react. Instead, embrace the truth that, of course, others may not agree with or understand your decisions, but if they're truly right for you, you will make them anyway. As a result, you will grow in confidence as you live a life that is more reflective of who you are, rather than reflective of the opinions of those around you. I've worked with clients who have spent years investing in a career route chosen to keep parents happy or impress friends. Well, you'll feel empowered as you say 'No more!'

- **Stronger identity and sense of self** How often do you profess to like something just because someone else is waxing lyrical about it? How keenly do you agree with an opinion or say a confident 'yes' while internally shaking your head furiously? As you choose to accept this truth, you'll stop contorting yourself to fit into other people's boxes. As you begin to speak out, to validate your needs and feelings, and to ask for respect, you'll nurture your self-esteem and see your confidence flourish.

- **Less need to seek validation** The more you are liked, the better you feel about yourself, right? At first glance there doesn't seem anything wrong with this. But accepting the uncomfortable truth that some people don't like you (and it might be nothing to do with you at all!) frees up worry, headspace, time and energy. As you begin to validate your own choices and feelings, no longer will your self-esteem take a swooping swan dive when someone fails to give you validation. You'll find confidence in the fact that you are a valid human being. End of. Everything else is subjective commentary.

- **Wave goodbye to people-pleasing** As you stop fearing the opinions of others, you can start investing your time and energy into the relationships that affirm and value you regardless of how much of yourself you give away. Enjoy more fulfilling relationships and honest conversations with those who care about you. For those people, 'like' is a response to *who you are* to them, rather than *what you do* for them.

- **Increased equality with others** Everything you do and say is a small but powerful statement of your worth. As you voice your needs and feelings, and ask for respect, you are making the statement that you are of equal value to others. Accepting the uncomfortable truth that some people won't like you is a leap towards equality.

- **Less defensiveness** In trying to protect your likeability, you may often feel attacked. Being misunderstood by others can prompt a desperation to explain yourself in order to ensure you are 'good' and liked in their eyes. As you accept that you cannot please everyone, you will no longer feel poised, living on the defence, ready to leap in to attempt to change the way people view and experience you. You will be able to relax into relationships and find more acceptance in the fact that you are not responsible for changing people's minds about you.

Which are the benefits that resounded with you? Maybe you'll find it helpful to reflect on the cost that denying the truth that you won't be liked by everyone has had on your life, your energy levels, your relationships and your self-esteem. I invite you to get off the people-pleasing hamster wheel. Sure, feeling liked by others can temporarily fill a void that exists because, underneath it all, you don't truly believe you're likeable. But just as a sweet snack satisfies before a sugar crash, chasing 'like' takes our self-esteem on a roller coaster of highs and lows.

But there's brilliant hope coming up. So yes, these days, if someone were to wildly gesticulate at me to get off my phone while I was actually picking crusty peanut butter off my jeans, I'd drive on and let it go. Life-changing. She didn't like me in that moment and that was okay. Not all of the time, but more of the time.

Five ways to accept being disliked

What now, then? You may have spent many years of your life, or even your entire life, trying to avoid the truth that some people don't like you. So how on earth do you challenge the habit of a lifetime? Here are five ways to start living with the glorious, headspace-bringing, boundary-affirming uncomfortable truth.

1. Take note of your internal chatter

If you believe that fundamentally you're acceptable, with all your flaws and tangled, messy secrets, then knowing that some people don't like you doesn't pack the same punch. This is the hardest nut to crack as the narratives and stories we tell ourselves, and have been told, can run deep. But it's a nut we can slowly crack, and one that comes with benefits that ripple throughout our lives, our minds, our decisions and our relationships.

One powerful way to accept displeasing others is to start noticing how you speak to yourself in the quiet of your mind. What tone does your inner dialogue carry? If it's impatient and critical, begin to follow it with a kinder alternative. In time, the compassionate voice gathers volume and the inner critic begins to fade. For example:

Dialogue: 'I can never please everyone. I said "no" when my brother asked me to pick him up from the airport because I had a shift at work, but now he's angry with me.'

Kinder dialogue: 'It's simply not humanly possible to please everyone! It's hard to disappoint my brother, but my responsibility is to be authentic, and to respect my needs and resources as much as I respect his. Sure, he's disappointed that he had to get a train, but if he finds it hard to respect my boundaries, it doesn't mean that my boundaries are in the wrong place.'

Along with becoming aware of your inner chatter, consider your behaviour. How are you treating yourself? Are you caring for yourself as if you respect and value yourself? Or does your self-treatment border on neglect or even abuse?

Let me ask you this: would you speak to and treat someone you care about in the same way you speak to and treat yourself? This is the greatest litmus test as to whether you're nudging your self-esteem upwards or downwards with each word and act. Begin to treat yourself and speak to yourself as you would someone you respect and care for, regardless of the discomfort you feel when you do. That discomfort will ease in time, I promise. As you treat yourself as someone who is acceptable and likeable, then you'll need less relentless external validation to tell you so.

When exploring this with a client, he recalled how when a friend stopped by for lunch, he took a moment to heat up some soup. My client admitted that when he's alone he usually snacks on 'sugary rubbish from the cupboard' for his lunch. We noted the vast difference between taking a moment to heat up some soup and sending his blood sugar on a roller coaster! The one speaks of value and kindness, the other of haste and lack of care.

Where in your life are you metaphorically eating sweets over soup? How might you treat yourself a little more as you would someone you value and respect? Begin making small changes and see your need for external validation soften as you start responding to your own needs with respect and kindness.

This topic deserves a whole book of its own, I know. I wrote a book called *Know Your Worth* that guides you towards important self-acceptance, and I recommend therapy for those who find self-acceptance hard to cultivate.

2. Understand how subjective 'like' is

I recognize that I wanted, no, I *needed* everyone to like me. But at the same time, I was fully aware that I didn't like everyone myself. In which case, isn't it a tall order to always be liked, when we don't always like everyone ourselves?

We know cognitively that we only see a sliver of people's lives, a mere snapshot of their front-of-house. Yet we consistently make sweeping judgements about others based on that small snapshot. We will delve into this truth in Chapter 7, but hold this in mind as you remind yourself quite how subjective 'liking' something or someone truly is. Can I wholeheartedly profess to love India, when I spent a mere month there at the age of nineteen? In the same way, can the conclusion you came to about a friend-of-a-friend being 'uptight' be a solid assessment of who they are? The conclusions we draw are only ever based on limited information, no matter how well we think we know someone or something. We see through our own limited lenses. We will never know the true depths, complexities, histories and mysteries others hold.

I don't like green tea. I never have and I don't think I ever will. I've told people this and they've suggested I try it in different ways – with lemon, with sugar, with milk – but, ultimately, it's not my bag. It's not that there is anything wrong with green tea itself. It's just that me and the tea aren't meant to be. I have other preferences and that's okay! Many people love green tea, ensuring it remains a permanent fixture on the shelves of homes and shops.

Next time you catch yourself thinking that you don't like something or someone, recognize that this is purely an opinion, reflective of your own personal likes and tastes. This helps challenge the power that we often give to 'liking and pleasing'.

A client of mine enjoyed one of those wonderful, life-changing 'Aha' moments as she recognized that to expect to be liked by everyone was a pretty humungous order when there were people in her own life she wasn't keen on. She recalled how she struggled with a colleague, not because she wasn't a nice person, but because their personalities and opinions clashed. It reassured her to understand that if someone didn't like her, it might well be due to something outside of her control anyway.

In the same way, if you're honest, you don't like everyone either. Often that's not a statement of their likeability, but simply proof of difference or preference. 'Like', therefore, is totally subjective. 'Like' is based upon preferences, narratives, experiences and opinions that most likely have little or absolutely nothing to do with you at all.

Someone once told me about their dislike of me, saying it was because I reminded them of their cruel cousin.

Apparently, I looked a bit like her. She didn't like me, yet the reason had absolutely nothing to do with me at all. So, whether someone likes or doesn't like you is mostly subjective, and it is the same with your assessment of others too. We give so much power to thoughts and opinions that, quite frankly, mean next to nothing.

3. Give your power to the right people

Make sure you have people in your life who know you well. If you don't, consider who those people might be and take small risks of vulnerability in opening up and sharing more of your truth and your story. Consider those people who know and accept you in full knowledge of all your flaws. The truth is that you are accepted by those people who know you best, therefore you are acceptable.

Write down the names of three people who know you well and, beside each name, write three things that act as evidence that the person accepts you. For example:

Kev, my good friend
– He checked in on me when Dad was sick
– He accepted my apology when I was short with him the other night

21

– He has seen me at my lowest points over the last few years and has continued to be a friend

Do you trawl reviews to help you decide whether to make a purchase or book a holiday? Would you trust a book review written by someone who hadn't read more than a paragraph? Would you book a holiday based on the feedback of someone who hadn't set foot inside the hotel? You wouldn't. Instead, you'd be more likely to seek and trust the reviews written by those who'd read the book front to back, or stayed in the hotel and eaten their way around it.

A client of mine was utterly floored by some criticism she received from a colleague. The colleague gave some feedback on a project that my client had been working on which sent her confidence into a 'tailspin'. Together we determined that the colleague had no idea of the intricacies of the project or how challenging it had been, and was therefore not in a position to provide accurate feedback. My client shared the feedback with her boss, who instead of echoing the criticism, praised her for how well she'd navigated such a difficult task. She recognized that the feedback from her boss was far more valuable and trustworthy than the criticism from her colleague.

I remember stalling a car on a roundabout and listening to the orchestra of horns around me as I scrabbled to restart the car with shaking hands. In that moment I felt the disapproval at my windows. They didn't know I'd been trying hard to address driving anxiety and was getting used to being behind the wheel again. They didn't know that, for me, even climbing behind the wheel was something I was proud of. They didn't know, but my good friends did. My friends' encouragement deserved far more power than the cacophony of impatient honks.

Remember this when you are giving a huge amount of power to the person who has chosen to dislike you, yet doesn't truly know you. It means little to nothing. Know to give that power to those who have read more than a page of the book of your life.

4. Don't push down feelings, process them

Feelings rise up in us as we respond to the world around us and the sensations within us. They move through our body or rest heavily on our chest; they feel like rocks upon our shoulders or sit like sludge in our gut. We so often quash them with criticism – 'I should be stronger, I'm a burden' – or invalidate them with gratitude – 'It's hard but I should be grateful, others have it harder.' Feelings are simply responses that give insight into the narrative and stories we tell ourself, both consciously and subconsciously, such as 'Someone not liking me means I'm unlikeable.' We live by these stories until we choose to change them.

Naomi, my client, had been invalidating her feelings for years. Whenever she felt like she'd upset someone, she would lose sleep night after night, dissecting the interactions she'd had with them and working out how to make it right. We spent our time together talking about what it means to upset someone and determining where her responsibility lay. I encouraged her to ask herself these questions:

Did I do anything wrong? 'I don't think so. From what I can recall I was kind to my friend, it's just that she seemed to ignore me when I caught sight of her yesterday.'

What story are you telling yourself? 'That I've annoyed her accidentally and she's mad at me.'

How can you challenge this story? 'Maybe she didn't see me. I could see how she is next time I meet her, and if she seems off with me, I could ask her if everything is okay.'

Where does your responsibility lie in this? 'It's my responsibility to be respectful, as I believe I was. I can ask her, but it's her responsibility to be honest with me if I have offended her in some way.'

Next time you acknowledge that you are experiencing fear or rejection in response to someone not liking you (or seeming not to), don't push the feeling down, get your torch out and shine a gentle light on it. Consider it with an enquiring mind and question what you could have been taking as fact. You might have been rejected, it might feel painful, but it's not a rejection of the entirety of who you are. Someone not liking you doesn't mean you're not likeable. Introducing an alternative narrative sends cracks through unquestioned stories and, in time, begins to powerfully shift how you understand and experience the truth of 'people don't like me'.

Keep observing feelings and questioning narratives, and you'll slowly reclaim the power that the fear of being disliked has had over you. It will become a truth you can accept, rather than one that prompts fear.

5. Push through fear and do it anyway

Feel the fear of someone not liking you and do whatever it is that you need or want to do anyway. As you begin to become aware of the things you aren't saying, doing or asking out of fear of others not liking you, start challenging yourself to do them and speak them out. See it as a social experiment and make a note of the times you step out and the world doesn't fall apart.

My client loved the gym. However, there was one person there who'd often spend ages talking to him. He would chat back as he wouldn't want to offend the woman, who seemed friendly without any sexual motive. But, in truth, he had limited time to spend at the gym and would leave feeling frustrated that he'd done more talking than exercise. He even considered moving to another gym!

We discussed what it might feel like to say, 'It's good to chat, but I'm limited on time so I'm going to head to the weights section, see you later.' He felt nervous the next time he went to the gym, but he forced himself to utter the sentence and, with a smile, off she went, leaving him to continue his workout. He also began to wear his headphones to create a sense of his own space and to mark a visual boundary. It felt transformative and enabled him to start speaking out in other situations too.

I remember being in envious awe of fellow commuters on the London Tube who would shout for everyone to move down the carriage to create space. I witnessed the murmurs and eye-rolls as people shuffled down. One day, with little standing space, I decided I would challenge myself to ask people to move down. With palms sweating, I shouted out. People moved. I felt the eye-rolls, but also the relief of those who gained the extra centimetres of space. Nothing bad happened.

As you step out and speak up, even with sweating palms and a shaking voice, even if the inevitable rumination follows soon after, you'll grow in confidence. You'll grow increasingly secure in the fact that you deserve your space in the world and people can handle you more than you considered they could. You'll recognize that we experience each other through the lens of our own experiences, and the best we can do is be authentic and respectful to one another.

So, next time you find yourself wishing you could speak out in order to ask for your needs to be respected, try it and see what happens!

Conclusion

Find a mantra, a short sentence, a reminder that prompts you when you catch yourself wondering or worrying about being liked or disliked. I like saying the two words 'So what?' to myself. This question carries an aloofness that encourages me to ponder whether it truly matters if someone agrees with my honest words or not, or whether they think my outfit clashes, or if they disagree with my deeply considered decision. Perhaps you ask yourself if they deserve that power over you, or remind yourself that, in living an authentic life as a unique individual, you simply cannot expect to garner approval from everyone.

Some people won't like you and the more you begin to live in acceptance of that, the more authenticity and confidence you'll enjoy along the way. Someone might not like you, but if you have two or three people in your life who see your dark and messy corners and like you all the same, then they're far better placed to make a call on whether you're likeable or not! So, lean into the truth that some people don't like you and preserve the energy you've ploughed into trying to ensure that the whole world gives you the thumbs-up.

JOURNAL POINTS

1. What has led to your denial of the uncomfortable truth that some people don't like you?

2. What costs have you faced in avoiding this truth?

3. What pledges can you make in order to begin living in acceptance of the truth that not everyone will like you?

Not being liked doesn't mean I'm not likeable

2.

I am Going to Fail

Diving headfirst into the uncomfortable truth

You will plough time and energy into something and it will fail. All of that work will come to nothing; in fact, it will come to far more than nothing. Along with failure, you have to wade through the feelings of disappointment. You may even feel dazed and confused as to why things didn't work out the way you hoped they would. You question your identity. What does this failing say about you? You thought it was so right, so how come you got it so wrong? Should you even bother trying again? Are you broken?

The collateral damage of failure can be immense. Failing to uphold a boundary in a relationship can find hearts broken and resentment boiling red and hot. Repeatedly failing to fulfil work commitments can lead to desperately wondering how the heck you're going to pay the bills. Medical failings can lead to grief and disillusionment.

You pin your hopes and expectations on an achievement and when it doesn't work it can feel like a rejection. Failure is a part of life, and we know that, but it's a hard truth to face if we're questioning whether we're the cause. It's hard when failure is followed by a barrage of self-criticism and shame. Did you just fail or are you a failure? You may look at the broken hopes around your feet and wonder how on earth you're going to pick yourself up and dare to risk failing again.

Fearing failure keeps us stuck in life, because as much as we like to think we know a lot about life, much of it is trial and error and most of it contains some risk. The more you try to avoid failure, the more likely you are to keep your life small, safe and limited. We avoid failure to avoid pain, yet actually, when you're coming to the end of your life, perhaps you'll realize that an even greater pain is to have limited yourself through fear.

Simeon began therapy sessions with me prompted by a general feeling of low mood. After getting a brief overview of his day-to-day life it was obvious that something was missing. He wasn't doing anything 'fun' or enjoyable. His days were mapped around work, TV and popping in on his grandmother. He would meet up with friends, but was feeling flat and lacking a sense of enjoyment in life. Simeon told me how, as a child and a teenager, he'd paint. 'I'd always have something on the go,' he said. I asked him when and why he stopped painting. 'I went to uni and studied fine art for a year. Suddenly my art was being scrutinized and graded, and I hated it. I spent less time in the art room and more time in the nightclubs, and dropped out after the first year.' Art had been therapeutic, creative and, most importantly, fun for Simeon, but when expectations and frameworks were placed around his art, he felt stifled.

The next time Simeon came to see me, he told me how he'd bought a canvas for the first time in fifteen years and had begun to paint. 'Art had become about passing and failing. I want to reclaim it for myself.' I loved seeing Simeon's well-being flourish as he reinserted this important piece of the jigsaw back into his life. He shared how he found it hard to remove all pressure and expectation from his artwork, but that he was finding it easier as the days went on to let his art be messy and expressive as he rediscovered what it meant to him.

In this chapter you will come to realize that failing and being a failure are two very different things. In accepting failure, you'll likely fail more, but you'll develop the tools to cope. And, like Simeon as he challenged his fear of failure, you'll experience more, because you'll recognize that failing doesn't need to feel like such a shameful thing after all.

My story

I have had to spend years unpicking a general, deeply embedded sense of failure. I used to set the bar of, well, pretty much every element of my life too high. To fail at something, whether it was clinching a job role or failing to explain my emotional state with enough clarity to be 'got' and understood, triggered feelings of shame. Failing worked to prove my flawed narrative that 'I am a failure'.

I felt like I had to strive so hard in order to feel deserving of the good things in life. I wanted to be the best employee, the best partner, the best mother. I believed that to be the best, I had to spend every ounce of energy and resource on getting everything right. It was utterly exhausting. I would regularly hit burnout, feeling depleted, low and wanting to retreat from the world. I'd pause in a teary heap on a Sunday afternoon, beating myself up for being a failure, before picking myself up, dusting myself down and pledging to try harder.

Only when I had kids and the call on my resources increased overnight did I find out, in a rather chaotic way, that ploughing all my energy into avoiding what I perceived as 'failing' was damaging me. I had to lower my unachievable bar in order to not be repeatedly criticizing myself for my own limitations . . . essentially my own humanness.

We fail a lot. Especially if our expectations are high. Accepting the truth that we fail isn't about being defeatist and not even bothering to try, it's about having compassion and grace for ourselves when things don't go how we wanted them to, so that we don't shame ourselves.

When we fail, compassion says: 'You tried. It's hard and sad that it didn't work out. What's the next step?' Shame says: 'You're a failure, why did you even bother trying? You were never going to be enough for that job.' Compassion enables us to move forward from failure by inviting us to see that there's a path beyond it. Shame leaves us feeling hopeless and unsure if we should try again.

So, if to fail is to learn and grow, why does the fear of failure have such a hold over us? Philosopher Nietzsche offers us this way of approaching failure: 'A thinker sees his own actions as experiments and questions – as attempts to find out something. Success and failure are for him answers above all.' He is encouraging us to see both our successes and failures as useful data in our attempts to discover things about life and ourselves, rather than 'good' or 'bad'. So how, then, can we move towards a new way of experiencing the things we often fear? In this case, our own failure?

Why deny?

We don't deny that we will fail. In fact, many people assume they will. Coming to acceptance of the truth that we will fail isn't about assuming we'll fail, but recognizing that it's worth a shot regardless of whether we do or not. And if we do? It's not the be-all and end-all . . . in the end. Failure can strip us and shape us and give us fresh perspective and learning that we wouldn't otherwise have had. This was the case for Simeon, who found that inviting art back into his life was all the more enjoyable because he proactively chose to let it be a messy learning curve.

Often, we are so acutely aware of failure that we don't even want to try to achieve the things we yearn for. You might assume that you'll fail at finding a partner who will love you, so you don't even look. You may assume you'll do a bad job of the project at work, so you procrastinate even starting, so much so that you end up putting yourself under huge pressure as the deadline looms.

Accepting that you'll fail, and fearing failure are quite different.

Accepting the uncomfortable truth of failure means knowing you'll fail at some things but also being confident that failing doesn't mean you are a failure. You recognize that trying may lead to failing, but there are things to be learned along the way, so it's worth a shot.

Fearing the uncomfortable truth of failure means failure prompts you to beat yourself up or shame yourself whenever you fail. Fear of failure has turned you into a master of procrastination. It feels safer to not even start anything or seek to achieve something rather than risk the feelings that come with failure.

- **You failed and it was awful** Perhaps you've failed in some way and the collateral damage felt too much to bear. Whether you were impacted practically or emotionally, it makes sense that you then avoid risking the consequences of failure again. Maybe your self-esteem and sense of worth are tied to success and, when you failed, your confidence took a painful battering. If you've been through something rough, you'll want to protect yourself from chancing it again.

- **You were taught that failure wasn't acceptable** Maybe when you were growing up, achievement was king. Perhaps your caregivers lavished you with love and attention when you did well at things, and you felt their disappointment when you failed. In this case, you learn that to achieve is to be accepted, and to fail is to risk rejection or separation from your caregiver.

- **Failure has become a statement** Failing is factual. You failed to fulfil the job role, you failed to bake the cake for the right length of time, you failed to remember your friend's birthday. Fact. But if you turn the fact of failing into a statement about your entire being – 'I am a failure' – it is deeply shaming. No wonder you're afraid of failing if your internal dialogue is bullying you.

- **Your self-esteem is rooted in your output** If how good you feel about yourself is totally dependent on achievement, success and output, then failing becomes a threat to your sense of identity. In this case, failing isn't just straightforward failing, it's a challenge to your very identity and your worthiness for love and good things.

- **We are measured by our success** We live in a culture that grades children from before they can even read or write, who measure one another in terms of followers on social media platforms, letters after names, square footage of houses, centimetres round a waist. No wonder we find failure difficult. We are taught that who we are is the sum cost of what we do, have and achieve. Failure is interpreted as a backwards step rather than a part of life.

As you've read through this totally non-exhaustive list of reasons as to why you might find the truth of failure a tricky one to face, I hope you recognize that you're not alone in this. Some may have leapt out at you and I encourage you to bear these in mind as you continue to reflect on the various costs that denying the truth of failure has had for you.

The benefits of embracing this uncomfortable truth

Before we look at the benefits of accepting the uncomfortable truth of failure, I want to acknowledge that there is one thing that holds my clients back initially from wanting to work on their fear of failure. Why should we come to terms with the fact that we will fail when it drives us to work harder and achieve more? Fear of failure has helped me get promoted at work because I've put in so many extra hours to prove that I'm up for the job. I've read and reread my work because I've worried that bosses will call me out on a mistake or criticize my attention to detail. I have tried extra hard in friendship groups so that I don't fail at being accepted.

So I don't doubt that sidestepping the truth of failure has got you to some good places in life. Me too. But if you're honest, wasn't most of that tainted by fear? Worry about the outcome? Worry about feeling like a schoolchild being told off by a teacher when you were found lacking? I truly believe you can be driven to achieve, with great outcomes, without the heart-racing fear of failure and all that it might mean to you. What is it that you'd like to achieve? Ponder that for a moment. Do you want to achieve stability, perhaps? Maybe you wish to climb the ladder at work and feel a little more stretched? Perhaps you simply want to find more balance or fulfilment in life or your relationships? What great things lie on the other side of trying (and sometimes failing) that act as motivators?

Now, hold these things in mind as you work through the benefits of seeking deeper acceptance of the inevitability of failure.

- **Embrace more opportunities** When failure is accepted rather than feared, it stops having quite so much power over the decisions you make. Perhaps you know all too well that an opportunity or two passed you by because the fear of failing made it feel safer not to even try to reach for it. Fear of failure can rob you of some of life's goodness, whereas acceptance of failure enables you to embrace more of the wonderful aspects of life such as adventure, deeper relationships and progression in your career. When you stop focusing on the risk of failure and instead start to embrace the inevitable risk, ploughing on regardless, your world opens up!

- **Procrastinate less** Procrastination is fear-based avoidance. You know there's something you need to do, but you just keep putting it off. As you begin to accept failure as a possibility, it becomes easier to get stuff done as there is less fear and pressure to get it right. You'll find yourself cracking on with the task at hand and more likely taking any failure in your stride.

- **Boost confidence and mental health** If your self-esteem is attached to whether you succeed or fail, then you'll be riding a roller coaster of feeling good about yourself when you experience success and questioning your worth when you fail. As your worth and your sense of identity become less dictated by how well something goes, then your confidence won't waver as much with failure. Your internal dialogue will become kinder as you won't criticize yourself as much when things go pear-shaped but will see it as a part of the process. Plus, with increased confidence and self-esteem, you'll be far more likely to do the things that nurture and support you.

- **Learn to welcome constructive feedback** Critical feedback and challenging words can be especially hard to stomach when you don't accept failure but fear it. As you feel more comfortable with failure being a part of your bumpy, upwards journey, appraisals and confrontation will no longer feel like a personal attack on your identity but an opportunity to discuss and grow.

Which benefit of accepting the ugly truth of failure made you most excited? Take a moment to reflect on the feelings you have towards failure and imagine how things might be different if it didn't hold so much power over your decisions and actions.

Five ways of coping with failure

How do you move from that place of fearing failure to accepting that it's a part of life and isn't something to be ashamed of? How do you stop limiting your progression by being more open to failure?

1. Validate your feelings

When you fail, there is often a sadness or frustration that follows. If you're feeling sad that your hopes didn't come to fruition, allow yourself to grieve the loss of that dream.

A client of mine spent our first few weeks together grieving the loss of a flat he had hoped to move into. He had failed the credit check. He spoke about how he had 'mentally moved into the flat since first viewing it' and had imagined his future there.

At first, he said he felt 'angry' with himself for feeling so annoyed at failing the credit check, but we acknowledged how the flat symbolized a fresh start for him. We explored how beneficial it was that he'd taken a proactive step and how it had uncovered some financial issues that he felt motivated to address in order to find another rental opportunity. In acknowledging the mixed feelings, he slowly moved past the anger he'd directed at himself and felt empowered to try moving forward again with fresh clarity on his financial situation.

Practise healthy ways of responding to the feelings that follow failure. It can be very tempting to ignore or numb them so you don't have to confront them. But then they sit beneath the surface, ready to pop out when you're next faced with a chance to risk failing. Feelings that we internalize and start to add to the narrative that failure is something to be ashamed of. So, speak them out, write them down, open up to someone, tell them about your disappointment and let them tell you about their failures too.

Imagine a stream running through a field. You can let the water flow or you can grab a bunch of sticks and stones and create a dam which holds the weight of the water back, under increasing pressure. The pressure builds up and then one day the dam wall buckles or the water spurts out of a crack sideways. This is what happens when we deny emotions: the pressure builds and eventually they will break through. Acknowledging your response to failure without judgement allows the emotions to move through you.

2. Create a kinder inner dialogue

The most important conversation you will ever have is the one that takes place in the privacy of your own mind. It feeds or starves your self-esteem and has a say in the decisions you make and how you respond to the world and failure.

Do you use shaming statements such as 'I am a failure, I am rubbish'? If so, address your critical inner dialogue. My client Lorna had never before observed her inner dialogue, so I encouraged her to listen to the way that she spoke to herself when she did something she perceived as 'bad' or 'not good enough'. The results were very telling and alerted her to how she had been viciously attacking herself verbally at any hint of perceived failure. Here are the steps I encouraged her to take. You will find them helpful as you begin to recognize your own internal dialogue.

Notice what you said to yourself in that moment: *I had forgotten to put the bins out and I told myself I was 'good for nothing'.*

Consider whether you would say these things to a loved one in the same scenario. If you did, what would the impact be? *Absolutely not! It's over the top and insulting!*

Do these words really carry truth? What impact might these words have on you? *I can see in my life that I'm capable at many things. So, it's not true that I'm 'good for nothing'. The words perpetuate the feeling that I can't get anything right.*

What might you say instead? *I could say: 'Oh dear, that's annoying. I've got lots on my mind so it's understandable that I forgot. I'll have to take a trip to the tip at the weekend and set a reminder on my phone for next week.'*

Of course, take responsibility where it is due, and if you've done something bad, then apologize, but don't let your inner dialogue become a bully that won't let you forget your failure. If you beat yourself up for something that wasn't actually your fault, or was an accident, then chipping away at your confidence and self-esteem through constantly criticizing yourself is a high price to pay. Note how you speak to and treat yourself when you fail, then imagine what a kind friend or coach would say to you. Say those words to yourself instead to help bring balance to your inner critic and to challenge any shame.

My inner chatter is drastically kinder than it used to be. I'd say it bordered on abusive throughout my twenties and early thirties. As a result, failure cut me deeply because it just affirmed that I was as rubbish as I feared and felt. Nurturing a kinder inner dialogue has taken a long time because, as for many of us, I have had to challenge a narrative and a harsh, critical voice that has been part of my inner world for all of my remembered life.

In time, as you recognize how you're talking to yourself and offer a kinder, balanced alternative, it starts to take hold. Gradually, the kinder words get louder and then they begin to integrate into how you respond to yourself automatically, I promise. These days, my inner voice is generally quite nice, like a firm, supportive mother who, instead of 'You're a failure', says 'Oh dear, that didn't go well, did it? What shall we do about it?' My feelings about failure, and therefore life itself, have changed for the better along the way as well. And in doing this, yours will too.

3. Remember all the times you've failed
This seems counter-intuitive, doesn't it? You're knee-deep in feelings of failure and I'm here encouraging you to dwell on other times you've failed. I'm not trying to pour salt into your wounds, but instead I want you to recognize how you moved on from those times.

Take a moment to write down a list of three to five failures. Beside them, write down some of your learnings from those failures. Consider what you learned about yourself, others, your work or life itself through that experience. Reflect on how that failure has helped shape who you are today. How did it dictate the steps you took thereafter that got you to where you are now?

My client Len found this process helpful. He had berated himself for years after a 'failed' marriage. The therapy he'd had immediately after his marriage ended had shone a light on how his lack of self-awareness contributed to the breakdown of the relationship, and he hadn't forgiven himself.

Before one of our sessions, he wrote a letter to his partner, accepting responsibility where it was due and apologizing. He read this letter out to me and that very act alone enabled him to begin the valuable process of recognizing that he couldn't undo the past, but now, with his increased self-awareness, he could enjoy a fulfilling relationship with his new partner. His ex-partner had moved on and he deserved to give himself permission to do so too.

You have survived each and every single failure so far. Of course, each failure will have had a different impact on your life. Perhaps you had to hear the words: 'I'm sorry, you didn't get the job.' Or maybe you've spent time grieving a painful relationship breakdown.

I run my own business and I've had to pull the plug on many different things along the way because they just didn't work out. The more I've walked through the motions of failure, the quicker I've begun to pick myself up. Of course, there are always exceptions to the story, and some failures feel like they come out of the blue and wind me, taking me back ten steps and leaving me questioning everything. But in the main my failings don't impact my identity as much as they used to. The more things I try, the more failures I'll face, but also the greater the outcomes too!

Listen to stories of those for whom failure was a significant part of their journey. You only have to read a handful of the stories of successful people to discover their past is littered with failings, big and small. It tends to be that one of the qualities of success is to learn to move past failure. Prompt yourself to find techniques and management skills if needed.

It's so true that some failures are more painful than others. But what our minds often do is lump all failure as difficult or traumatic if we've had a couple of bad experiences. Knowing that your brain does this is a helpful tool because recognizing that fear is stopping you, and that not all failure is horrendous, offers an opportunity to press on with this knowledge in mind. Hearing that failure is a part of people's stories helps challenge this narrative too and can even turn some failures into empowering, instructive stepping stones that become a part of your own story.

4. Know that failure isn't full rejection

I'd like to share with you a new way to consider failure. Imagine you bought a brand-new tent. You open it to discover that one of the poles has arrived bent. You take it back to the store. It looks like you're rejecting the whole tent, but there was nothing wrong with the rest of it; in fact, it was pretty darned perfect. The issue was with a single part. It's not that the tent failed you, it just meant it wasn't fit for the specific purpose you needed. In the shop you find another tent, and ask to swap it.

When failure feels like it cuts deeply, it's likely because you are interpreting that failing as a reflection on the entirety of who you are as a person. If it feels like failure is saying 'You're a failure' rather than 'Oh dear, that didn't go well', then it needs reframing.

I encouraged a client of mine to drill a little further into the detail next time she found herself proclaiming that she was a failure. She found it so helpful to turn a vast, shaming statement into one that felt clearer and more factual. She turned 'I failed at work' into 'I lost my calm. I'd benefit from working on my patience', moving her from a place of shame in which she felt stuck to one where she identified an area for growth.

Here are some examples of other ways to reframe 'I'm a failure':

- *My skillset failed to match up with the job spec. I need to develop my skills.*
- *Parenting is tough. Perhaps I need some support.*
- *I'm sad the relationship ended. I need to allow myself to grieve.*
- *That was tough feedback. I'll talk to a friend to help me process it.*
- *That really hurt, but I know I didn't do anything wrong.*

Can you see what I'm doing here? I want you to begin reframing that sense of 'I'm a failure' into a tangible statement that focuses on the actual thing that failed, didn't work or didn't add up. Failure isn't a full rejection of who you are but some feedback about a part of you or something you've done. If you don't get the job, it's feedback. It's not that you're all bad or below par or undesirable. It's that you don't match up, or didn't gel with the interviewer, or don't have the right experience; or maybe even something that wasn't about you at all, like catching the interviewer on a bad day.

5. Keep your standards fair

If I ask you to jump a hurdle, and I set it at Olympic height, I'm setting you up for failure. If you give it your all and you fail, is it because you didn't try hard enough, or is it that the bar was simply set far beyond your physical capability?

Johnny, my client, discovered that the bar he set for his own fitness hadn't moved since he was an athlete at college: 'I used to run 100m in 17 seconds. It's like I have it in my head that I have to stay at that level of fitness.' He acknowledged how important fitness was to him, but how he battled consistent feelings of failure at not being able to maintain the numbers he used to reach in his teens. We discussed at length how his targets needed to be amended to suit a man of forty-five with a busy job. It took him time to accept his changing levels of fitness and ability, but with the help of a personal trainer, he set new goals that challenged him while giving him the opportunity to feel empowered when he hit age and lifestyle appropriate targets.

Ask yourself this: where in your life do you think you might be failing because the bar you set for yourself is too high? How might you readdress the aim, the bar, the boundary in order to reduce the pressure and take into account your humanness and limited resources? When you're not setting yourself up to fail quite so much, facing the truth that you will fail sometimes, doesn't seem quite so jarring.

My story resonates a little with Johnny's. I love to work out. It is an absolute favourite tool for my mental, emotional and physical well-being. I used to follow workout plans that told me exactly what I needed to do, and would feel like a failure when I couldn't tick everything off. Perhaps I'd had a rough night, wasn't well or some work had come in last minute. Either way, the narrative I had that I needed to stick to every single thing on this plan didn't leave much margin for life and its curve balls. These days, I just see what I have in the tank each day and, if I do follow a plan, I'm much more accepting of 'failing' to follow it to the letter. I have added humanness into my expectations and it has made things so much more enjoyable.

Perfectionism and needing to do well in order to feel confident can be a driver to set the bar of expectation that little bit too high. You may find that striving for excellence keeps you motivated and doing well in areas of your life but at what cost? Burnout happens when we continuously push beyond the limits of our own resources. Make sure when you are setting goals for yourself that you are taking into account your humanness as you do.

Conclusion

I'm hoping to have sent cracks through how you see failure, shaking it up a little bit. My main hope is that you'll recognize where failing leaves you shaming yourself and will approach it in future with a more open and enquiring mind. Don't be disheartened if you find it difficult to break the habit of self-criticism whenever you fail, it takes time. But aim to look critically at what happened, rather than to criticize yourself. Looking critically at something means to analyse and observe it in order to draw conclusions; it's not the same as criticizing, which focuses on the negative.

I could add into every single section of tips to seek therapeutic support if needed. Sometimes we have been shamed at a time in our life by someone important to us. We were made to believe we were failures long before we could rationalize that we had simply not been able to meet the (often too high) bar that someone set us. Recognizing this is always a useful step forward in coming to terms with failure.

You fail, but you're not a failure. You might have done something bad, but you are not bad. You might have got something wrong, but you are not wrong.

JOURNAL POINTS

1. Write down any shaming statements or narratives that you have used towards yourself. Now rewrite them in a more subjective and kind way.

2. What is your internal dialogue like? Is there someone you might model your more compassionate voice on?

3. Note down some of the times you've failed and moved on from.

———

Failing doesn't make me a failure

3.

I Will Hurt People I Love

Diving headfirst into the uncomfortable truth

You do and say hurtful things. You always have done and you always will.

Sometimes you hurt someone intentionally. You want to. They might have hurt you and you just want them to know how it feels. You probably know them well; you know their weaknesses and their regrets so you can use just the right words to inflict pain. When you hurt them, you feel both pleasure and shame.

You also hurt people accidentally. People have winced inwardly because something you've said has pressed upon a sore place within them, and they've gone away with your words resounding in their ears. People have felt unimportant to you or dismissed by you because of the way you've treated them. You're not even aware of how what you did or said changed the way they feel about you. Perhaps someone is not sure as to whether to bring it up or not, or whether they're being too sensitive.

If you knew how you'd hurt them, you'd feel mortified. You didn't mean for it to come across like that. You simply forgot to invite them to the event, or you really didn't see them that day when you walked down the street, or you truly overlooked the fact that their dad was seriously unwell while you ranted about an argument you'd just had with yours.

You've hurt people in both small and relationship-changing ways, through misinterpreted words, sarcasm, forgotten details and accidental betrayals. You could move through this world with the best of intentions and you'd still hurt people. You could exhaust yourself trying to weigh up how everything you do and say might come across to someone, and you'd still hurt people.

I love the words of Japanese writer Haruki Murakami in his novel *South of the Border, West of the Sun*:

[. . .] ultimately I am a person who can do evil. I never
consciously tried to hurt anyone, yet good intentions
notwithstanding, when necessity demanded, I could
become completely self-centred, even cruel. I was the
kind of person who could, using some plausible excuse,
inflict on a person I cared for a wound that would never
heal.

Isn't that true? That we can be the kindest intentioned
person, yet when we come under threat, we so often seek
ways to protect ourselves, which may mean harming
others in some way. It's human survival, everyone for
themselves. It sure can be ugly and messy sometimes.

My client Kay told me how she would 'forever feel bad' for
discussing a detail of one friend's life with another friend.
'My friend shared with me that she had an eating disorder.
A few weeks later, I was talking to a mutual friend of ours
and I disclosed this information to talk about how we might
best support her. I totally see now how I was betraying my
friend in sharing this information, but it truly came from a
desire to work out how to help her.'

Kay was devastated when her friend called her up in anger
and told her how betrayed she felt. While Kay apologized

profusely, explained and also acknowledged how inappropriate it had been to share this, her friend was unable to forgive her and the friendship has been ruptured for months. Kay said, 'In truth, I also shared it because the truth felt like a big secret to carry, and I felt a bit helpless so also wanted our mutual friend to share in it with me.'

Sometimes, like Kay, we wish we'd navigated things differently, but our choices carry a cost that, regardless of how sorry we are, we cannot put right. There's the uncomfortable truth. We will hurt people we care about. I wonder what thoughts and memories are surging up as you read these words. Perhaps some specific situations that sit like spiky burrs in your memory or give you an acidic feeling in your gut. Maybe you're feeling a wave of regret or shame as you think back to particular things you've done or said, or a sense of helplessness at the fact that you will hurt people regardless of how empathetic and compassionate you are.

My story

Knowing that I'd potentially hurt someone used to feel excruciatingly painful to me. It was like a red-hot poker jabbing directly into the core of my belief that I was bad. I'd ruminate over words I'd used, searching for a reason why my friend might have replied in that way, or why they'd spoken to everyone in the room yet turned to address me last. If someone seemed upset, withdrawn, irritable, I'd assume it was my fault. Nobody could be around me having woken up on the wrong side of the bed or having a tough day without me wondering, 'Are they being short with me? Are they cross with me? What have I done?'

I'd try desperately to investigate whether I'd upset someone. I'd shower them with chatter and attention, looking closely at their face to frantically determine whether they were being cold or responding in the way I'd expect them to. I'd fire questions at them like a detective to try to tell whether I'd upset them. If I knew them well enough, I'd ask, 'Are you okay? Have I upset you?' To be honest, as I write this, I think I must have been a bit exhausting at times, needing regular reassurance from those around me, reading hurt into simple bad moods. I imagine that in some cases I may well have annoyed people, thus creating a vicious cycle and fuelling my rumination.

In all honesty, though, on the flipside, I'm pretty good at hurting people. When I feel attacked or misunderstood, I am articulate, I am quick to think and I can sharpen my words like arrows before throwing them straight into the epicentre of vulnerable places. In moments I feel threatened by those close to me, I can be cleverly, deftly hurtful. Perhaps I think my feelings have been dismissed or misunderstood and I want to create those feelings in the other person so that I don't feel so acutely alone in my own. I feel hurt and I want to hurt back. In those moments of fight or flight, I pick up my sword and I jab it into vulnerable places. I twist words that were spoken to me in moments of honesty, I get my shovel and dig up past regrets that have long been apologized for to prompt pain and shame so that I regain a sense of power. I don't do this often, and I don't like it. But feeling emotionally cornered and vulnerable has most of us scrabbling to use what we can in order to fight or flee the extremely vulnerable feeling. Once the dust has settled, I am left feeling ashamed at the lengths I went to and the words I threw like grenades, creating collateral damage that now needs clearing up.

Accepting the uncomfortable truth that I will hurt people has been another slow-burning, life-changing acceptance.

I have begun to take responsibility for the things I am responsible for, and have started to choose, very consciously, to let go of that which is not my responsibility. For example, I can treat others respectfully, but if they are harbouring anger or hurt because of me, and I'm not aware of it, then it's their responsibility to either talk to me or let it go. If I recognize that a relationship has shifted and I'm not sure why, I can ask if everything is okay. If they choose not to talk about it, I have fulfilled my responsibility. If I have hurt someone, whether on purpose or unintentionally, it is my responsibility to apologize, whether the apology is accepted or not.

This acceptance has come about by holding a microscope over my deepest pains, caused by those in my life who have hurt me most through not treating me or supporting me in the way I had hoped they would, or in a way that the role they played in my life dictated they should. Be it the teacher whose responsibility was to guide me, who in fact bullied me. Or the drunk patron who followed me home after my waitressing shift and tried it on with me. His responsibility as an adult was to respect my boundaries as a human. Perhaps it was the family member who was so consumed by grief that they weren't able to be present for me in the way I needed them to be in my childhood.

I have recognized that, in the main, it was their own unprocessed pain caused by how they themselves were treated that challenged their ability to give me what I needed when I needed it most. Their behaviour wasn't actually about me. The pain they caused me was a by-product of their hurt and not a reflection of my worth. In some cases it was a person's clouded ability to see my worth, because they couldn't identify their own. I had wrongly felt responsible for someone else's behaviour. As I recognized this, the hurt became less like that spiked burr and more of a smooth stone that built part of my story.

In the same way, I realized that I need to take responsibility for therapeutically addressing my own pain, so that I don't hurt others as a result of it.

Why deny?

You'll know that you've hurt people as you've moved through life, accidentally and on purpose. Perhaps there's a relationship that couldn't be repaired after those harsh words were thrown, or, as in Kay's case, a decision that was made and can't be unmade, and you've carried a sadness around ever since.

So, it's not like you're denying the truth that you can hurt people, but when you fear hurting others or you take responsibility for other people's pain where it's not due, it comes at a cost. Let's look at some of the things that might have led to you feeling this way.

- **You take responsibility that isn't yours** If you often assume things are your fault somehow, it's likely you fear hurting others, so much so that you do anything you can to avoid causing others any kind of pain or discomfort. You filter your words, deliberate over your actions, and if someone seems upset, you automatically question what you might have done to hurt them before you even question whether it's you they're upset with.

  If this resonates with you, it may be because as a child you had to internalize your feelings in order to maintain a relationship with a caregiver. Or perhaps you were cared for by an adult who struggled to take responsibility for their own behaviour and therefore would place blame elsewhere. Maybe you assumed a parenting or caring role with your caregiver as they struggled to be the 'adult' in some way. Any of these scenarios may have taught you that to continue an important relationship with a caregiver and maintain survival, you had to assume the role of peacemaker. The dynamics that exist in childhood to ensure survival can often continue on into our adult lives when they go unchecked.

- **You were blamed for someone's feelings** When you've grown up feeling like the cause of someone else's pain, you may have had to navigate the fact that your caregiver consistently seemed hurt or offended by you. In order to preserve such an important relationship, you come to believe that you are the problem, and you do what you can to make them happy. You move through life with the sense that to upset someone risks causing painful disconnection.

- **Fearful of confrontation** If someone has hurt you, you may find it hard to talk honestly with them about it. Perhaps you swallow down the hurt and try to continue as if nothing has happened, or you'd rather withdraw from or avoid someone than talk about it. Equally, if confrontation feels vulnerable and scary, you may try to do everything within your power to avoid causing someone hurt.

- **You've been hurt** Maybe you've been hurt in the past, the pain felt intolerable and the relationship changed somehow. When a relationship has been ruptured, it can feel tough to believe that another relationship might be able to withstand messy, human hurt, or the weight of your honesty and emotion. Your emotions and opinions may well take second place to the comfort of others if you have previously felt emotionally or physically unsafe as a result of expressing your authentic feelings. It's important to know that if someone hurt you as a result of your honesty, because you placed a boundary or demanded respect, it doesn't mean that you shouldn't have done those things; nor does it mean that others won't respect you. For some reason, they weren't able to, and it may well be zero reflection on you at all.

Which reason for feeling fearful of hurting people jumped out at you most? Hold that in mind as you identify some of the costs. It might be surprising quite how much this fear has impacted your relationships, but don't forget, awareness introduces a fresh element of choice. And when you're aware of the choices you have available to you, that's when you can start making different decisions and seeing a shift in your life and relationships.

The benefits of embracing this uncomfortable truth

When we spend our lives trying to avoid hurting others, we undoubtedly hurt people a little less because fear has us treading extra carefully in situations we otherwise wouldn't think too deeply about. I have watched my partner write text messages with such care and thought. He takes a lot more time than me. I'm sure my hasty, slap-dash messages have resulted in more confusion or misunderstanding along the way than his ever have. I send a lot of messages to friends and family, and if I spent time considering each sentence and word and how they might be received, it would be so time-consuming I probably wouldn't bother sending them at all.

That's just one tiny example that came to mind about how worry can cost us time and energy, but let's delve further into the many benefits of embracing the uncomfortable truth that you will sometimes hurt others regardless of how hard you try not to.

- **No more fearing the elephants in the room** When you fear hurting others, it can be tempting to avoid conversations about certain things in order not to cause confrontation. Perhaps they've hurt you somehow, or there has been a misunderstanding. However, when you recognize that your responsibility is to be authentic and considerate in how you express yourself, rather than to control how the person receives your honesty, there no longer needs to be any awkward elephant in the room. The truth is that we often attempt to leave the elephant standing there to preserve the relationship, but of course the relationship is acutely impacted by that which goes unspoken. The equilibrium we're trying to maintain is only surface level. So when we no longer fear the elephant, and find ways to address it, we can be truly authentic with one another. If the relationship can withstand the truth, then it will be all the richer and more enjoyable for it.

- **Enjoy new depth of relationships** Vulnerability, openness and honesty are ingredients of deep, rich relationships. To feel close to someone, you must feel safe to be yourself with them. When you fear hurting others, you may hold back from having certain conversations or expressing your needs and feelings. As you embrace this uncomfortable truth, you will benefit from deeper and more authentic relationships as you find new ways to be more 'yourself' with others. Allowing yourself to be truly seen by another person is a powerful way to feel validated.

- **Grow in confidence in having difficult conversations** The more often you do something, the more confident you get at it. If you currently believe that difficult conversations usually end painfully, no wonder you avoid having them. As you challenge that belief, you'll begin taking the risk in talking about what needs to be talked about. In time you'll realize that, yes, some of those conversations won't go as you hoped, yet some of them will be empowering and productive. Maybe they will actually clear the air and make way for a deeper level of relationship.

- **Enjoy more equality in relationships** When fear stops you from sharing your thoughts, feelings and needs, you are denying your equality in a relationship by believing someone else's feelings are more important than yours. As you step out in being more open and valuing your own experience of a relationship as equal to the other person's, you will benefit from more relationships that feel equal and two-way, and therefore more mutually enjoyable and beneficial.

- **Find it easier to apologize and move on** Because you fear hurting others, when you do hurt them, or you believe you have, you find it incredibly difficult to move on. In facing this uncomfortable truth, you recognize that all you can do is apologize and attempt to reconnect with the other person; you cannot determine how they respond to your offering. You'll need to spend less time and energy with any continued apologizing or 'making it up to them'. This means that the issue won't impact the relationship for longer than it needs to as the other person doesn't need to keep offering you reassurance in order to restore your confidence that all is forgiven. But also, if the other person will not accept your apology, it means you can find a way to move on or grieve that relationship rather than relentlessly trying to change their mind.

All of these benefits involve refusing to deny yourself somehow, don't they? You are choosing to no longer deny yourself richness and depth of relationship, confidence, authenticity or headspace free from rumination. I wonder what you would add to the list as you've moved through it and pondered the benefits?

Five ways to live with hurting those around us

You've identified that you worry about hurting people and it shapes how you interact with them. You're now aware of quite how much avoiding this uncomfortable truth impacts your relationships, so how on earth do you loosen your grip on it? How do you get to a place where you accept that you'll hurt people along the way through life? How do you strike a balance between wanting to be a good person – because there's nothing wrong with that – and fearing getting it wrong all the time? I've got some ideas.

1. Work on confidence

Low confidence and the fear of hurting others come hand in hand. You're a good, imperfect person who sometimes gets things wrong, whether you mean to or not. It's the truth of your humanness, and the result of living alongside others with their own histories and idiosyncrasies. We all view each other and interpret the world through the lens of our own experiences.

When you are often holding yourself back or choosing not to express your needs, you are putting your authentic self on hold. When you consistently make yourself small, simple and needless in order to avoid upsetting people around you, you are stopping yourself from growing in confidence.

Think about how often you ask friends and family how they are. In the same way, begin asking yourself the same question. I encourage my clients to ask themselves 'What do I feel? What do I need?'

Frannie, one of my clients, would come into our session each week seething with frustration at her partner. 'Every day, she leaves her mug on the worktop above the dishwasher. It's like she expects me to put it in there. Why can't she just take one second to put it inside? Every time I mention it to her, she just tells me to chill out and says she'll do it later so I've stopped asking.' After a few weeks, we decided to explore this dynamic in more detail. I asked Frannie to identify what she felt and needed.

'I feel like she doesn't care what matters to me. I know it's not the be-all and end-all to her as to whether the mug sits there all day or not, but I work from home and I like the kitchen to feel tidy when I work. I always have done.' As for the need, Frannie identified that as 'I need to feel like I matter to her. It doesn't take long to shove the mug in the dishwasher, but it matters to me.'

Frannie found it helpful to identify that, in the end, it wasn't 'just a mug'. The mug being left on the side was symbolic of the bigger theme of needing to feel like her preferences mattered to her partner, no matter how 'silly' they might seem. In light of this, Frannie was able to have a more in-depth and productive conversation with her partner about the wider picture of 'the mug' and how simply placing it in the dishwasher was not just a pernickety request but a way to honour Frannie's working environment and an opportunity to demonstrate care.

So, next time you have a feeling that would benefit from a bit of detangling, ask yourself: 'What do I feel? What do I need?'

Asking yourself these questions is a way of both evaluating and valuing your emotions and needs, whether you choose to verbalize or act upon them or not. Valuing yourself builds confidence, little by little.

2. Know where your responsibility lies

When you've upset someone, think about what you feel responsible for. Grab a piece of paper and list the things you have assumed responsibility for, rightly or wrongly. This is an example from a client session of mine:

I feel responsible for:

- *The fact that I said I couldn't go to my friend's fortieth birthday party. He feels let down. I've said I'm sorry but I feel to blame for that.*
- *The fact that he is probably paying for my meal at the party, so will be down on cash.*
- *The fact that my mum feels bad that I'm not going to his party because I'd agreed to pick her up from the hospital instead.*
- *The fact that I feel like I've let my friend down and made my mum feel guilty.*

Now, let's explore this list a little, and perhaps your own list will benefit from my reflections.

Steve, my client, prioritized picking his mother up from hospital over attending his friend's birthday party. This decision sat in line with his own value of 'family first' and was an authentic decision that felt right for him. His friend feels let down. That's okay, he's allowed to feel however he feels in response to Steve's decision. However, Steve has apologized for the fact that he won't be there. Steve has not done anything wrong or unkind, he has simply navigated the circumstances in line with his own values. If his friend chooses to allow the feeling of being let down to impact their relationship, then that's a shame. He may instead choose to accept the fact that Steve wanted to be there for his mother and allow himself to feel both disappointment at his friend's absence and compassion for his circumstance. Steve cannot control which path his friend takes.

As for Steve's mother's guilt, it shows us that she perhaps finds it hard to accept kindness from others, or that it is tricky to navigate the shifting dynamics in which her son has an opportunity to mother her. Regardless of what is fuelling her own guilt, Steve has made a choice willingly, and her guilt is a reflection of her own internal world rather than anything Steve needs to work to relieve her of.

You are responsible for respecting other people and for respecting your own boundaries too.

If you have hurt someone, you are responsible for apologizing, but you can't control whether or not that person accepts your apology. This is the difficult bit, right? It can be painful when the other person doesn't want to or isn't ready to repair the relationship. I often work with clients who are journeying through the twelve steps in Alcoholics Anonymous (or similar). Step 9 is about making direct amends where possible. Often clients encounter people who aren't willing to accept apologies or don't wish to reignite relationships or return to old hurts. If this resonates, I encourage you to allow yourself to feel sad that they aren't able or ready to accept your apology. Let them know that you're there and willing to talk should they want to.

If you hurt others through holding a boundary that keeps you safe and well, then it doesn't necessarily mean there's a problem with your boundary or your perspective. Consider where your responsibility lies, and if you've taken responsibility for your part in the story, then it's up to the other person to take responsibility for theirs.

Your responsibility:

- Taking ownership where needed
- Apologizing appropriately
- Respecting and communicating your boundaries with kindness

What you can't control:

- Whether or not someone accepts your apology
- Whether or not someone chooses to respect your boundary
- Whether or not someone chooses to take responsibility for their part in the rupture or dynamic

It's hard when other people choose not to repair the relationship or respect the boundary you have set for yourself. It's also tough when someone might find ways of continuing to 'make you pay' for your mistakes or keeps bringing up your failings. This can feel rather persecutory and makes it difficult to repair and move forward.

It might be that the other person is hurting or battling disappointment and for their own reasons is unable to move on. You are not responsible for fighting these battles for them. Choose to forgive yourself even if the other person isn't able to. You can opt to let yourself off the hook after you've apologized, even if they can't. This means that you can find your own way to move forward. It can feel like a tough pill to swallow when a relationship doesn't feel the same again and you may feel a grief for that loss.

3. Learn to have difficult conversations

Learning to have difficult conversations is such a skill for life! If the fear of hurting others is what holds you back from voicing an opinion or a hurt of your own, practise with those you feel safe with.

Ella worked up to having one of these conversations within our sessions together. She acknowledged that she felt fearful of addressing her stepmother's criticism of her parenting, which seemed continuous and underhand. We spent time discussing the ways she could address this, which ranged from writing a letter to setting a date for a coffee to share how the sarcastic comments her stepmother made felt critical and unsupportive. Ella settled for a more informal 'can we have a quick chat' option, and rehearsed a simple way to begin the conversation: 'I find it hard to talk about these things, but I pick up on the small comments you make about how I choose to parent and I want to know if you're finding it hard to respect the parenting route we've chosen.'

Ella said that the conversation, on the whole, went fairly well, although she noticed her heart rate rocketing as she instigated the chat. The opening line of 'I find it hard to talk about these things' felt both honest and empowering for her, and meant that she didn't cue herself up with the pressure to get it completely right.

When I was trying to grow in confidence in difficult conversations, one of the most helpful things I did was to be honest about how hard it was for me: 'I find this so hard to talk about, but our relationship is really important to me, so I owe it to you to be honest about how I've been feeling so that we can find a way to move forward.'

Taking the risk to have difficult conversations and choosing to work through conflict leads to stronger connections and deeper relationships. With each difficult and honest conversation you have, you learn that the right relationships can withstand your honesty and requests to have your boundaries respected. Perhaps you could ask a friend for advice on how to approach the difficult conversation you need to have, as talking to others may well help you find a new and creative solution. Sometimes it's also helpful to catch up with that same person after you've had the conversation by way of debriefing.

I remember one specific difficult conversation that didn't end in the way I'd hoped. The other person did not take my honesty very well at all. They felt hurt and confused. I took a risk and it didn't pay off. It made it evident that our relationship couldn't withstand the disruption of scratching beneath the surface, and instead of deepening our relationship, it deepened the confusion and sense of misunderstanding. Fortunately, I have had many other difficult conversations that *have* ended well, and taking the risk of vulnerability has resulted in richer depths of understanding, so I know that even though it may not always end well, it is always worth it.

Take a moment to consider some of the difficult conversations you have had over the years. Reflect on these points:

- How did that conversation go?
- What did you learn from it?
- Did you take responsibility where you should have?
- Did you take responsibility that wasn't yours?
- How did that conversation shape the ongoing relationship?
- Did the other party take responsibility where they should have?
- How did this impact your confidence?

Difficult conversations involve stepping out and taking risks. It can feel nerve-wracking at first, and you may do it with your palms sweating and your voice shaking, but do it all the same. Remember that there is no such thing as a perfect conversation and you can only be true to yourself and respectful to the other person. Each conversation that goes well will build your confidence in being your authentic self. Each one that doesn't go well is an opportunity to learn, to review where your responsibilities lie and perhaps an invitation to grieve.

4. Address your own hurts

Imagine you're standing on a busy train station platform. You are packed tightly like sardines, your arms pressed against the arms of people next to you. Nobody bats an eyelid. You shuffle forward an inch as people try to board the busy train and your bag brushes my arm. 'OUCH, watch out!' I shout at you. You sense my anger and feel guilty as you see me rub my arm.

I'd had a flu jab that morning. My arm was aching and when your bag brushed my arm it sent a deep wave of pain running down towards my fingers. Was that your fault? In truth, you triggered a pain that was already there. Your bag didn't cause my pain, it alerted me to it.

When we don't address our own hurt, we're more likely to hurt others, whether intentionally or unintentionally. Unaddressed pain, hurt, anger, grief and resentment spurt out sideways when we keep the lid on. As much as we would like it if they stayed neatly inside, they don't: the pressure builds up and they become more urgent.

If we don't acknowledge our own pain, then other people are more likely to be on the receiving end of our wrath. Unacknowledged trauma and painful feelings get triggered and we can find ourselves shunted into a fight-or-flight response when anything happens that is reminiscent of the original situation or touches on the original pain – whether it has anything to do with it or not.

One of my clients, as a child, was sometimes called 'stupid' by an adult she looked up to. 'You stupid child' would be spat at her sporadically, and she'd feel like 'I must have done something terrible'. In fact, she concluded that 'I must be terrible'. For many years thereafter, hearing the word 'stupid' directed at her in any context, even if it was totally flippant such as 'Well, that was a stupid decision', would trigger a visceral reaction. In a flash, she'd feel like a child being told off and a wave of shame would flood her.

The more my client told me about this adult, the more we understood as to why they were so harsh. They had been mistreated as a child and not given the tools to consider how their responses to others might impact their relationship. While you too may be able to explain why a person has hurt you, it doesn't necessarily excuse it. Why am I telling you this? Because you will be more easily triggered by the actions and words of others if you're already in pain. Find a way to process and give voice and acknowledgement to your pain.

Here are some steps to help you do this:

- Explore where the true responsibility lies, and if you've taken responsibility for behaviour that was not your 'fault'.
- Choose to let that narrative go (and keep letting it go when it surges back).
- Have therapeutic conversations with those you feel safe with or visit the Helpful Contacts section at the back of this book.

Allow yourself to grieve relationships that have been fractured by hurt. As you move through that loss, then the truth that you will hurt others even when you're simply being authentic to your feelings and needs feels less unnerving.

5. Get comfortable with unanswered questions

A client of mine recalled how one morning, before seven a.m., she had leapt to google the name of a strange illness she'd read about on social media but never heard of, and also searched to find out what the weather was doing that day. She had been trying to reduce her screentime and it struck her that neither answer actually mattered to her. What seemed to matter most was the feeling of harbouring an unanswered question. We acknowledged how, in our current digital age, no question ever need go unanswered.

I relate, do you? One rare, quiet Sunday afternoon, my mum and I did the crossword in the paper. It was everything we could do not to grab our phones and find the answers we were struggling with.

When it comes to people, though, it's not so easy. If you've hurt someone and you don't know why, or how, or you can't understand why they're not able to accept your heartfelt apology, it's hard to not know the answers. Perhaps they don't even have the answer themselves as to why they feel the way they do. Sometimes the answers don't have anything to do with you at all.

Learn to sit with the wondering. Maybe you're feeling restless at not knowing what your friend has done over the weekend and your finger is hovering over the social media button. You know that, if you click, time will disappear like sand between your scrolling fingers. Maybe you want to dig, dig, dig by throwing questions at someone, despite feeling that their guard is rising by the second.

The next time you find yourself scrabbling for answers, ask yourself this: would the answer really benefit you? Or could you challenge yourself to sit with the wondering?

If someone is cross with you, and you've asked them if they're okay only to receive the retort 'Yeah, fine', then sit with the wondering. If you worry that you've offended someone with a misplaced joke, but they seemed unruffled, then sit with the wondering. If you wonder what is going on with the news, but you've had your fill and know it will feed your anxiety if you plough through any more articles, then sit with the wondering.

Our brains are created to wonder. Every piece of information we bombard it with needs processing and filing somewhere in our grey matter. This consumes energy and headspace. Learn to sit with the unanswered questions and you'll slowly learn to feel a little bit more comfortable with the unknown. Fulfil your responsibility and let the questions settle. It's a difficult practice, but it's possible.

Conclusion

I believe we all have an 'inner child'. If you haven't heard that term before, it's a theory that I have found so helpful and acknowledge within my clinical work. Psychologist Carl Jung is thought to have coined this term, which acknowledges that we all experience inner feelings and emotions that seem childlike. Your inner child is the bit of you that has never and will never fully grow up. If we don't acknowledge our inner child's feelings and needs, they may hold a huge amount of power over our adult self. For example, a recovering addict I worked with shared this, which I feel illustrates the inner child concept beautifully:

'My inner child wants to use all the time. He lives in the moment. He says, "Sod the repercussions, I want the drugs and I want them now." Only when I started to separate out my inner child from my grown-up self did stuff start to change. My adult self wants to be sober. I know what is right for me and my life and relationships. I realize that my inner child wants to act out and doesn't care for the consequences. My inner child feels any hurt or stress and wants to numb it. In my early days of recovery, I used to talk to my inner child all the time, reassuring him that we didn't need to use, we needed to ride out the feelings. Honestly, it changed my life.'

We can all feel young and vulnerable sometimes. It's the little voice that yells, 'I'm tired, I don't like this, I don't want to do this,' while the adult part of you pushes on. You are constantly parenting your inner child. Do you recognize when you do this? Whether you give yourself encouraging pep talks or you criticize yourself for being so ridiculous, it's happening.

So, when your inner child is all at sea because someone seems to be hurt and they feel at fault, turn towards that young, vulnerable part of you and offer words that will ground instead of shame: 'Let's say sorry for what happened' or 'You didn't actually do anything wrong, I'm not sure why they're feeling cross. Perhaps they're having a rough day.' This tack can be life-changing for those who feel taken back to childhood relationships when people are displeased or hurt.

Don't abandon yourself. You have needs, feelings and opinions that have value. The more you take risks in expressing these, even when your toes are curling in your shoes, the more you will learn to recognize what is your pain and what is someone else's. This realization has changed my life and I hope that, in time, it might change yours.

JOURNAL POINTS

1. What fuels your fear of hurting others?
2. Where have you taken responsibility that was not yours to take?
3. How have you abandoned yourself in the pursuit of avoiding hurting others? How might you reclaim your voice?

I can control **my choice** to apologize. I cannot control **how someone receives** the apology

4.

I Can't be Fully Present All the Time

Diving headfirst into the uncomfortable truth

Your focus isn't always in the here and now. Life-affirming moments will pass you by and your head will be elsewhere. You will spend time with the people most important to you and you will leave feeling like it was all a blur, barely remembering what happened let alone what you said. Your head was in a work drama, your heart was at home on the sofa.

You'll miss firsts, you'll miss sunrises, you'll miss shooting stars tearing through the sky because you were busy gazing at the dirt around your feet. You'll lose loved ones and curse yourself for not inhaling every moment of their presence while you could. You'll feel sobered and you'll pledge to make the most of life for evermore lest you miss out on the things most precious to you. But hours later your mind will be pondering things that don't matter, you'll waste time, your focus will shift towards the to-do list yet again.

What does it actually mean to 'be present' anyway? You are there in body, always. You can't have half your body here, in the moment, and half of it in tomorrow. You are here, right now. As soon as you are aware of the moment, you are in the moment. You might not be inhaling it or walking around in a Zen-like state of gratitude-fuelled joy, but your focus is on what's in front of you. I think by 'being present' we are alluding to the fact that we are neither looking backwards nor forwards, we are focusing on what we're doing, feeling or seeing, whether we wish to pause time or hit the fast-forward button.

This could easily get rather deep and philosophical, but I'd love you to think about what meaning you apply to the term 'be present'. Who is ever focused on the moment all the time? Who can be? How can anyone move through life and function as part of society if their focus is only ever on the very moment in front of them?

Your attention isn't always in the same place as your body. It can't be. What would get done? What would get planned for tomorrow? You'd live for each day, like a baby, like an ant, just moving from moment to moment, totally immersed in the feelings and drives that arise, with little regard for anyone else or the impact one decision might have on the next moment. Sometimes this would be wonderful but what about the moments that feel excruciatingly painful or dull? What about those moments you're wishing away rather than savouring? They'd feel never-ending without the perspective that the past and future bring.

The more we recognize that we won't and can't always have our focus on the moment in front of us, the more we alleviate the pressure we place upon ourselves and the guilt and shame we feel when we realize we've missed things, memories and people along the way. By accepting the uncomfortable truth that you will not always be present, you're actually freeing yourself up to recognize when the choices arise to focus on the moment in front of you. By acknowledging that you will inevitably miss valuable moments along the way as you whizz by in a rushing daze, you won't be too full of regret to see the wonder in front of you that's still there for the taking.

This feeling of regret was all too familiar for my client Ned, whose brother died in a road traffic accident. 'We were meant to go and watch a football match the week before, but I cancelled due to the worst hangover ever. It has haunted me ever since. I will forever kick myself that I didn't go, and that the last time I saw him I was distracted by an issue at work. I feel like I can never say no to any opportunity to see a friend or family member, just in case, and that I must be a hundred per cent present when I'm with them.'

Together, we acknowledged Ned's grief and regret, and how cruel life can be. We spoke about how his brother's accident was a tragedy, not an everyday occurrence, and questioned how realistic it would be for Ned to never decline a meet-up or expect himself to feel fully present when he's with others. He admitted that he would exhaust himself and that the expectation to be fully present would pile pressure on to social occasions.

In this chapter we will relieve some of the pressure and guilt that come with expecting ourselves to be more present in our lives. Ironically, in accepting the uncomfortable truth, you may well find yourself engaging in life even more so.

My story

I remember when my little sister's cancer took hold, and the care she received moved from trying to sustain her life to ensuring that she had the most comfortable end to her life. We loaded the car with food and packets of drugs and went away to spend a weekend together as a family. It was a 'holiday' of sorts, but we knew it was our last as a unit of five. Every trip thereafter would feel like a piece was missing.

One morning I woke early, keen to start the day. I went to wake my sister and I paused to stare at her sleeping face. I felt starkly aware that I'd soon be navigating life without her. I swore, in that moment, to make the most of every second I had left with her.

Despite my intentions, within seconds of her waking we were arguing over something or other. Perhaps fighting over who had eaten both boxes of chocolate cereal from the miniature variety pack. Days later, I yelled, 'I hate you!' in the way kids sometimes do. For years, I looked back on that with deep shame. The thing is that in both of those instances I was truly living in the moment, responding to what was happening in front of me.

Sometimes I recognize that the pressure I place on being present is actually pressure to enjoy a moment. As a parent, I get told to 'Enjoy every moment', I see quotes set over smiling faces saying 'You get eighteen summers with your kids, make them count'. Can you see how these words taint the very moments in front of us with shame and guilt? How much can we truly let our focus fall on whatever sits in front of us when we have a voice yelling at us to enjoy it? This is exactly what Ned and I touched upon in our sessions as he spoke of pressuring himself to make the most of every moment with his loved ones.

I recognize how I often get caught in the thick of things, things that don't matter. I sometimes catch myself on my phone while my kids are vying for my attention. My mind wanders elsewhere in moments I've been looking forward to for months. I crave holiday time, yet struggle to switch my mind off from work. I meet up with an old friend, yet I'm barely listening to what she's saying.

When I notice my focus is elsewhere, I am suddenly out of autopilot and faced with a decision to refocus. I can continue on autopilot, with my mind on a million things, or I can take in the scenery. As soon as I recognize I'm on autopilot, I have a choice. As I've begun to accept the uncomfortable truth that I simply cannot always be present, I've actually become more intentional.

In his *Notebooks 1935–1951*, Albert Camus shared his thoughts on being present and the pressure we place upon ourselves to experience everything fully: 'You will never be able to experience everything. So please, do poetical justice to your soul and simply experience yourself.' What I take from this is the encouragement to remove the pressure to experience every moment fully, and to place the focus instead on living authentically and embracing our unique experience of whatever lies in front of us.

As I've removed the pressure to be present in every moment, I've been freed up to experience more gratitude. As with many of these truths we're exploring, the less I try, the easier it becomes. Go figure!

Why deny?

Why is the call to be present such a big one in our society? And why do we put so much pressure on ourselves to enjoy the moment? I believe it has become such a focus because our minds are constantly engaged in a powerful tug of war. Focusing on the moment is the antidote to everything that the digital world is pulling us away from. So let's look at why it's tough to take the relaxed approach to being present that comes with accepting we simply cannot be so all of the time.

- **The relentless buzz of technology** Technology invites you to stay switched on. Your attention is the commodity that has a price attached to it, whether a business has paid to have you thinking about their product, the algorithms are drawing you towards certain paid-for editorial or ads, or someone is paying for your clicks and likes. You are pulled towards technology like a sailor lured towards rocks by the siren call of the mermaid. You feel robbed of time and attention, and so you pressure yourself to focus on that which truly matters.

- **Boredom is becoming extinct** You want to be more present in your life, but you are uncomfortable with boredom. Only years ago, you'd stand in a queue and your eyes would roam into the spaces, faces and places around you. You'd be reminded of the bigger picture of life in seeing the community around you and the natural world above you. These days, we are taught to avoid boredom by filling our minds with words and images from screens almost surgically attached to the palms of our hand. Boredom inspires creativity, it leaves space for emotion to ebb and flow, and for dreams to be pondered upon. Boredom is the fertile soil in which our minds can expand; we need it yet are constantly tempted away from it.

- **We are encouraged to avoid difficult feelings** There are so many ways to avoid feelings. You can numb them with substances, dulling heartache or stress with drugs and alcohol. You can work, work, work, leaving little space to rest. You can drown out thoughts with music streamed into your ears or back-to-back box sets. I have spoken to clients who have feared that if they stop, slow or pause, they will drown in the tears they've never cried, or ignored needs will suddenly fight for attention. No wonder the call to be present, all the time, feels like an overwhelming prospect.

Your time, focus and attention are one of the most important commodities you have in life. Companies literally do what they can to buy it, and it costs them a lot. We feel it pulled away from us and we believe the antidote is to grab it all back and hone our focus in on the moment.

The benefits of embracing this uncomfortable truth

Here are some of the brilliant benefits you'll experience as you take steps to embrace the uncomfortable and guilt-relieving truth that you'll never be fully present in your own life.

- **Less exhausting perfectionism and greater self-esteem** Rejecting the guilt-rendering belief that you are missing out on life as it whizzes by means you'll be less likely to be consumed by perfectionism. Why? Because when you focus on what you believe you've done wrong, or fixate on the areas you feel you're lacking in, the response is often to try harder. You lean into the belief that if you manage to achieve being present, then you'll feel less guilt or grief at what you would otherwise have missed. As you stop pursuing something that you'll never succeed in, you'll sidestep all the related self-esteem-harming self-criticism.

- **Relinquish the guilt that you're not present** Guilt follows when you believe you've done something wrong, or somehow fallen below the bar of your expectation. When you recognize that you'll never truly absorb every single moment of a special occasion, or make the most out of seeing an old relative, then that pang of guilt won't follow. Guilt and shame sit in the gap between the standard we set for ourselves and the reality of what actually happens. As you stop beating yourself up for not being fully aware of every special (or mundane) moment, your self-esteem will benefit and, ironically, you'll be more likely to embrace those moments more fully without that pressure to drink it all in.

Unless you live in a secluded location where you are cut off from society, with only a babbling brook and cooing birds for company, you're going to have your attention pulled in many directions. Even then, in that Zen-like fantasy, you may be concerned about where your next meal comes from or preoccupied with pangs of longing for the people you've left behind in your pursuit of perfect presence.

Five ways to live with not always being present

So, if you can't always be present, does that mean you shouldn't pursue it at all? Does it mean you should not bother to focus on the moment, the wonder or the challenge in front of you? Should you allow your mind to run untethered into the future or let it wander in memories of the past?

No, it's worth seeking to be present and choosing to focus your mind on what is in front of you when you remember to. Often, when we look back through the days of our life, it's those moments that act like photographs because we've made an effort to absorb a little more of them. Those moments punctuate our memory when everything else becomes a blur. In those moments we can absorb the joy or navigate the challenge wholeheartedly. So here are five tips for seeking presence, while at the same time letting go of any guilt that might result from forgetting to do so.

1. Sometimes survival is your gift

When you're moving through a tough season in life and all your focus is on putting one foot in front of the other, you're in survival mode. You're not going to stop to gaze in awe at the flowers as you move by them because your focus is on the moving alone. If you're on an aeroplane and the pilot yells at you to buckle up and brace yourself, you're not going to choose that moment to peruse the duty-free brochure.

Gina began our first session in floods of tears, sharing how she felt she had neglected her friends since being in a car crash. Not only had she been physically harmed when a drunk driver crashed into the side of her car the previous month, but her confidence on the road had been reduced to nothing. 'I used to see my friends all the time, but when I'm with them, I just can't talk like normal, my mind is elsewhere. I'm worried it will impact my relationships.'

Over the following sessions, I reassured Gina that the trauma she'd encountered was so very recent and it would take time for her mind and body to process and heal. I encouraged her to remove the pressure to be as chatty and invested in her relationships as she would usually be, and see this as a season in which her friends could support her. Her priority, I encouraged, was to go gently on herself, remove pressure, and to consider what emotional or physical needs her friends might be able to support her in. She concluded that her friends could come round individually for coffee, instead of pressuring herself to meet them in a group, requiring a journey. She began to recognize that, for now, she was in survival mode as things stabilized again, and in time her confidence would grow, both socially and on the road.

In a different way to Gina, I also pressured myself to continue as normal despite a challenging time. For a long while I felt a deep sense of shame that I'd had postnatal depression. There are reams of photos on my camera roll which I can barely remember taking. I was in survival mode, caring for two young children while feeling like the lights had been switched off in my mind. I didn't want to inhale the moments with my baby, I wished them away because I struggled to see past the pain. I now realize how, in that season of my life, focusing on the moment wasn't the best gift I could give my family – focusing on survival was more important.

The more you guilt yourself for not being present and enjoying the moment in front of you, the less motivated you'll feel to seek or accept any support that you might need to help you out of survival mode. Plus, it's so helpful to know that if you're going through a traumatic time or you encounter a traumatic experience, your mind can actually intentionally reduce how 'present' you are able to feel in order to try to limit the impact of the trauma.

So, if guilt arises because you've struggled to feel present in tough times or found it hard to see the good stuff in front of you, consider these three things and note down your responses if you feel able to:

- How do the expectations you have of yourself mentally/ socially/physically reflect the challenge you have been through?
- What guilt are you carrying? Remind yourself that you are doing the best you can with the resources you have and choose to let that guilt go.
- Give yourself permission that, for now, your focus should be on placing one foot in front of the other and accepting the support you need.

2. Choose not to judge yourself for how you feel
With the pressure to be present, often comes the pressure to feel good things about what is happening. It's okay to find hard things hard. It's okay to find boring things boring. It's okay to be overwhelmed by overwhelming things. Why do we apply pressure to ourselves to experience otherwise? You're having a human response

to your circumstances in any one moment. Let go of guilt for not always revelling in everything or for wishing the days away.

'My mum has dementia. I feel guilty every time I struggle to spend time with her,' said Dan in one of our sessions. He shared how his mother would sometimes be verbally insulting, or would often forget who he was, telling him to get out of her house. She would repeatedly ask the same questions and, as much as he tried to remain calm and patient, he'd find his responses becoming brusquer. 'I felt like I had to make the most of every minute I had left with her as I could see her slipping away every time I saw her. I mean, physically she was there, but at the same time, there were less and less windows of the "her" that I knew.'

Dan's story illustrates how much pressure we can place on ourselves not only to be present but to enjoy the moment we find ourselves in. In truth, not every moment is enjoyable. Some of them are boring, some painful, and some are downright traumatic.

It can be so tempting to label the emotions we experience as 'good' or 'bad', 'desirable' or 'undesirable'. Actually, they're just feelings that arise, peak and subside. They say nothing about how grateful or not you are, or how capable or not you are. Dan's emotions were frustration, hurt and confusion, but he also shared with me feelings of fear as to what lay ahead for his mother, and grief as he recognized he was losing elements of her character that were familiar and special to him.

Try to avoid judging yourself or applying meaning to the feelings that arise by categorizing them. Some moments are messy and hard, and you want to escape them, and that's okay. In recognizing the feeling that has risen up in response to what you're seeing or experiencing, you're actually choosing to be present.

I have been so interested to discover that the less I judge myself for messy emotions, the more I'm able to focus on what's happening in and around me. When I am not pressuring myself to feel grateful and present all the time, ironically, I am more present because I'm not beating myself up for feeling overwhelmed or irritable, or trying to numb my feelings.

The next time you're criticizing yourself or trying to override how you feel in response to the moment you find yourself in, use this powerful tool: say, 'Right now I feel [insert your feeling], and that's okay.'

3. Use gratitude to bring balance

The truth is that you cannot always be present. Your focus is being called in so many different directions that you can find your head spinning. It's hard to allow your awareness to settle on what's in front of you when everything flashes for your attention, proclaiming equal urgency. If you often find yourself bogged down in the mundanity of life or your thoughts feel scattered, if you recognize that your mind is running ahead, fuelled by anxiety, into a future that has not and may never happen, use gratitude to anchor yourself.

Gratitude is the simple act of noticing what is in front of you that is good and real. It is like dropping an anchor down into the moment and seeing it for what it is. What is good in the moment you're in? The soft curve of the sofa, the sight of someone you love and are glad has a significant place in your life, the smell of the meal you're about to eat, the glance at the trees poking their way above the buildings you see through your window?

In the pandemic, a lot of my therapeutic work was around sharing how to use gratitude in a way that didn't invalidate emotion. One client talked about how she would often feel overwhelmed as she darted between her job in the local food shop and trying her best to home-school her son: 'I tell myself that I should be grateful I can still work as I have friends who are self-employed and now have no income. When I feel scared about bringing Covid home to my son and partner, I tell myself that I should be grateful I'm in a shop and not working in a hospital.' We recognized that every feeling she deemed 'ungrateful' would prompt this gentle kind of self-shaming.

In attempting to always 'look on the bright side', she was choosing not to acknowledge those very real and valid feelings of overwhelm and worry. It was a survival skill many of us leant on at that time.

Gratitude has undoubtedly shifted my day-to-day outlook on life and brought more balance to my emotions. Our mind often focuses on the negative, whereas gratitude invites us to also look at what is good and going right, be it the steaming mug of tea, the time spent with a friend or the bluebell shoots peeking up through ground which was recently frozen. It's about recognizing the wonderful alongside the messy, the beauty alongside the pain. However, gratitude should come with an asterisk and some small print. It should say: *Used well, gratitude will change your life and bring fresh balance to your emotions. Please don't use it as a stick to beat yourself up with or to invalidate valid feelings.* Gratitude is finding the awe and wonder alongside the darkness, not instead of it. It's about welcoming acknowledgement of the good alongside the tough, rather than totally ignoring and denying all that is hard.

I will leave you with my favourite gratitude tool. Turn 'I've go to' to 'I get to'. Let me show you how this works. Consider a mundane task such as taking the bins out. 'I've got to take the bins out' is full of drudgery and boredom, a task anyone rarely gets excited about. It's a job to tick off.

Let's turn that statement into an 'I get to' to draw your attention to the privileges within it: 'I get to take the bins out using my healthy legs that serve me so well each day, outside a home that keeps me safe and warm. The bin is full of rubbish, remnants of food we have afforded that has energized our bodies, which will be taken away by a refuse collector.' All of these things are privileges we tend to take for granted and overlook until they are challenged or lost to us.

4. You are always in the moment, but your focus can't be

Now, consider this. You are always IN the moment. I know that seemingly contradicts this entire chapter in which I'm saying 'You cannot be present all the time'. In truth, you are physically present, here, reading this book. You are fully in this moment, but your mind may be wandering to your to-do list, or perhaps you're glancing at your watch, thinking about heading out.

You are always in the moment. Your body, your mind, your soul are in this very moment, right now. You can't physically leave your body behind and head off into tomorrow, or lie in bed with your mind sitting at your desk. But your attention won't always be in the moment. You need to be thinking about later on, or your mind may want to reflect on something that happened yesterday or last year by way of processing it. Things happen in the now that prompt memories and feelings related to things you've experienced in the past, as well as things you hope to or are worried about experiencing in the future.

For me, and for many I speak to, it's a pressure to try to be totally present in a focused, fully appreciative and aware state. We see it as an antidote to the speed at which life seems to move past us. If we are present, we don't miss anything, we have fewer regrets, and we will never look back, as we often do, and wish we'd made the most of what we had when we didn't fully realize how precious it was. Now, that is the kind of presence we cannot maintain.

Meditation was a much-beloved tool for my client Ben. In fact, the way he spoke of its power within our sessions spurred me on to engage in meditation more often. 'I meditate a lot,' Ben told me. 'But the most important type of meditation for me isn't when I'm sat against my sofa for ten minutes in the morning. It's when I'm in the shopping queue or on the bus. It's when I'm with my mates or walking my dog. What I do is focus my attention. That's all. It's that easy. My mind is busy and scattered, but I just choose, when I remember, to focus my attention on something in front of me. My dog's wagging tail, my mate's rough, skilled, gardening hands as he holds his pint glass, how the woman in front in the queue is tenderly holding her husband's arm.' He shared how those moments, in the busyness, were meditative to him. Not the constant focus on everything going on, but the choice to grab his own attention, harness it from wherever it had scattered and direct it to linger on something in front of him.

So, as Ben acknowledges, the mind is busy, your attention is demanded and all over the place. It's not your fault that you can't stay focused on the moment in front of you, it's not psychologically possible to do it for long. Even the most seasoned meditation teacher will find their thoughts wandering to lunch at the rumble of their stomach.

However, there are ways that you can punctuate your day with presence. So consider this tool: find your flow. I'm not talking about yoga (although that's another great tool to help you feel more grounded), I'm talking about a state you may find yourself in organically or which you can choose to enter. I bet you've already experienced flow-state many times. Think back to when you last felt like time just disappeared because you were so engaged in what you were doing that someone could have rung the doorbell and you'd have barely noticed. Perhaps you were doing something creative or playing sport. Everything outside of that activity paled into the background. This is your flow-state. Those are wonderful moments, incredible at reducing stress levels and nurturing your resources.

Another way to move our focus into the present moment is to slow down intentionally. I often catch myself running around my own home, racing down the stairs as if I'm being chased. It adds to the feeling, during stressful times, that I am living on a treadmill where the speed is set a touch too fast for my legs and I can't find the button to turn it down.

When you move or talk unnecessarily quickly, your nervous system believes you're under threat somehow and prompts a release of stress hormone. You're not going to be noticing a sunset or truly listening to the words someone is speaking when you're in stress mode. Slow your movements and speech when you're stressed in order to calm your body and slow your mind.

Before I got married, someone gave me a tip. 'The day will go by quickly, in a blur,' they said. 'Make sure you remember to stop and really look at the scene a few times throughout the day so that you take a mental photograph.' I remembered this advice, and at one point in the evening, we walked up the stairs and stood on a wooden balcony. From there we could see all our friends and family dancing and talking. Almost fifteen years later, this is the clearest memory that I have.

So, every now and again, pause and remind yourself to take a mental photograph. Look around a little more intentionally, inhale deeply. Notice the sounds, sights and sensations both inside and outside of you. Look, really look at the people around you and notice nature, if it features. If the scene is a good one, whisper 'Wow', and activate a sense of awe and wonder. The things we remember are often the highs and the lows, but there is so much beauty in the mundane too that gets missed along the way.

5. Don't put joy on hold

Do you ever realize you're playing the 'when, then' game? *When I get that job, then I'll be happy. When I meet the right person, then I'll address my overworking. When I get to the weekend, then I'll actually slow down.*

Don't put life on hold. Don't kick the can of your needs down the road until another day, another season, another goal is achieved. Life is happening now, and drawing our attention to it is how we prevent it all from passing by in a blur.

A client of mine had put off addressing his depression because he assumed the heavy cloud would quickly recede when he reached the peak of his career. 'I remember the day I finally made CEO. I stood on the mountaintop of everything I'd worked towards for thirty-five years,' he said. 'I'd reached the pinnacle of my job. I was devastated because I still felt the darkness in my head. Where could I go from there? I thought it would be better to be dead.'

The 'when, then' game had prevented my client from getting the support he needed. The depression didn't abate with the promotion, just as we might not get fresh confidence from some good feedback, or benefit from waiting until midnight strikes on the first of January to address a self-sabotaging habit. Through our sessions, talking and finding tools for my client's depression, he began to feel empowered to make a number of lifestyle changes he'd been delaying. His quality of life improved and his feelings of depression abated.

The 'when, then' game stops you from getting what you need that will make your life more pleasant in the now. Who knows what tomorrow brings? Nothing is certain. As the truth of that settles in more comfortable ways throughout this book, hopefully you'll start recognizing even more so how life is about the now.

On a piece of paper or in a journal, write down some of the things you've been delaying or holding off until you reach a certain target or day. And then consider how it might benefit you to challenge that! Perhaps you decide not to wait until the weekend to slow down a bit, but incorporate more restful moments into your weekdays. Perhaps it's something as simple as not waiting until a 'special' day to use that bottle of fancy shower gel gathering dust in the cupboard. Maybe you pledge to catch up with your old friend now, instead of waiting until life eases up a bit.

Yes, of course you have to plan, yes you have to think about tomorrow, but where are you holding off joy, where are you holding off seeking support or going after something good? If you can, don't put it off until you've reached a goal, a certain life stage. You won't always be able to focus on the present moment in front of you, but 'now' is the only place you can truly live and experience your life. 'Now' is the only time that actually exists.

Conclusion

Have you ever noticed how there are often two streams of dialogue in your mind? I think of them as the parent and the child. My child dialogue rarely shuts up. It is observant, thoughtful, reactive, emotional and easily distracted. It ruminates and worries, and chatters when I want it to be quiet. Do you recognize your own child voice? As your child voice chatters on, you can become frustrated that you're not present or focused.

That chattering voice isn't who you are. 'So, who am I, then?' you ask. You are the one listening to it, you are the one guiding and noticing it, calming it or asking it to 'hush' (or belittling and criticizing it, if you tend towards a critical inner dialogue).

The adult dialogue in my mind is the more measured one. A little more thoughtful. This is the one that speaks back to my distracted, buzzing child voice, urging it to calm, refocusing it, parenting it. Some may recognize these parts of themselves as the rational and irrational brain, or the emotional and the logical brain.

So, when you criticize yourself for not being present, remember that you're always there. You are always in the moment, it's just that your focus isn't. Give yourself a break, cut yourself some slack.

Your busy mind hops between the past, the present and the future. Sometimes you hold all of these different states in mind at once. You are noticing the present and it gives you a bodily sensation linked to a memory.

You are everywhere and you are here. You are always here. The moment you recognize your buzzing mind is elsewhere, you are fully present. The moment you conclude, 'Eugh, this is hard,' you are present. The moment you pause and proclaim 'Wow', or urge yourself to survey the scene in front of you, you are present. The second you draw attention to the feeling of someone's skin under your fingertips or the shallowness of your breath, you are present. The instant you recognize that your thoughts are racing or listen to the pitch of someone's voice as they tell their story, you are present.

JOURNAL POINTS

1. What does it mean to you to 'be present'?

2. What stops you from being present?

3. Having considered where you're playing the 'when, then' game, what action will you take now, rather than waiting?

———

The moment I recognize that my mind is elsewhere, I am present

5.

Life isn't Fair

Diving headfirst into the uncomfortable truth

Bad things happen to bad people. Bad things happen to good people. Children die, random attacks happen. Innocent people get sentenced to death row while the guilty roam free. Less qualified candidates achieve the promotions, leaving the ones who really deserved the job in the lurch.

Unless you're always winning, everything goes your way and things constantly fall into the perfect place for you, then you're probably very aware of life's unfairness. Perhaps this truth washes over you or maybe it cuts you deeply. I'm betting a bit of both, and all that lies in between. You let a board-game cheat win because they're younger than you, but you lie awake with red-hot rage searing through your veins because someone publicly undermined you to make themselves look good.

Life is generally a survival of the fittest. And, even then, it's not a fair race. People have different advantages thanks to where they were born, what families they were born into and what physical attributes they have. We are dealt a hand of cards before we even arrive into this world. Curve balls swipe even the healthiest, fittest and most academic individuals, and sickness and cancers don't discriminate. If life's a race, it's not a fair one. But it's not to say that we aren't all competing in this unfair game.

You're aware that you're always at risk of being overtaken by someone somewhere. If you weren't striving and competing in some areas of your life, would you be where you are in your job? Would you even have a job if you had chosen not to compete against others in order to get offered it? If you have a partner, perhaps at one point you realized you weren't the only one in the running, you had to prove you were going to be a good partner, and in doing so, probably took a look around you to see what that looked like. The awareness of life's unpredictability and unfairness is what keeps you making decisions to better your life and to ensure that the good things within it stay there.

But also life's unfairness will have made you angry. Perhaps you are harbouring a painful sense of injustice because someone treated you badly, or perhaps a colleague took ownership of your success and got promoted ahead of you. Maybe a child you care about is being bullied or you bear the scars of someone else's pain. You may be grieving a loss that felt unfair, someone who died too early or through a medical mistake. It's not fair.

Can you imagine a fair world? Nobody would fall in love with anyone who didn't love them back in the exact same way, and relationships and friendships would only break up when both people felt mutually happy to do so. People's pay grades and the fruits of their labour would be directly related to how much time they spent working and how hard they tried. Nobody would die before they'd completed their bucket list and were grey, old and ready to resign. It would never rain on anyone's special day, unless they wanted it to. But what if someone else wanted sunshine? What if the farmer prayed for rain? Oh no, I'll stop there. You can see how this gets tricky. In his book *Don't Sweat the Small Stuff*, psychotherapist Richard Carlson wrote:

> **One of the mistakes many of us make is that we feel sorry for ourselves. Or for others, thinking that**

life should be fair, or that someday it will be. It's not and it won't. When we make this mistake we tend to spend a lot of time wallowing and/or complaining about what's wrong with life. 'It's not fair' we complain, not realizing that, perhaps, it was never intended to be.

I personally believe that fairness is worth striving for. Lives, cultures and structures have been changed for the better in pursuit of fairness. However, as with all of these topics we are exploring, it is nuanced. Sometimes life's lack of fairness in the circumstances we encounter is out of our personal control. In those instances, recognizing where to loosen our grip on the fight for fairness can be a gift to ourselves, saving us precious headspace and energy, while also allowing us to validate our feelings.

'Dad left me and Mum when I was three months old. He had an affair, and has never tried to get in touch with me since,' my client Anoushka told me. 'I tracked him down on social media to discover that he has a whole other family and, despite the fact that Mum and I struggled for money, he seems to be rolling in the stuff.' Anoushka was a high achiever, who shared that her motivation for doing well in life was to 'stick two fingers up at Dad and show him how I could do just fine without him'.

Over our sessions together, Anoushka contemplated her burnout, and recognized how her rage-filled desire to prove something to her dad was exhausting her and negatively impacting her sense of well-being and mental health. Anoushka slowly began to accept the uncomfortable truth of life's unfairness, and gave herself permission to feel her grief and sense of abandonment along with her very present anger. In doing this, in time she felt able to redirect her energy from relentlessly proving herself to her father to instead seeking her own enjoyment and balance.

Nobody ever said that life was fair, so why does the truth feel such a tough pill to swallow? If life isn't fair, why does acknowledgement of this leave us tossing and turning in our beds, fantasizing about how we might ensure someone gets just what they deserve . . . and not in a good way?

My story

It didn't take me long in life to recognize that, no matter how good I was, bad and sad things would happen to me.

Perhaps I'd thought that being good was some sort of protective shield against the world, that if people liked me then they'd be kind to me.

I still remember my utter confusion when a friend I made at school was repeatedly unkind to me. She'd lie outright about things I had said or done in order to ensure that I was told off by teachers and sometimes even my own parents. She would tell our friends tales about things that had not happened in order to encourage them to be cruel to me as well.

I was deeply confused. Instead of stepping away from the friendship and investing my time in other people, I tried harder to win her over. Surely the reason she was being cruel was because I wasn't good enough for her? She'd drop the cruelty and we'd become good friends for a short while, until the cycle began again.

That's just one example of unfairness, but I can remember throughout my life hearing bad or sad news and feeling a lightning jolt of shock that such a thing would happen to 'them' or to 'us'. Just like Anoushka, it made me feel vulnerable to acknowledge that life isn't fair. Goodness is no impermeable shield to bad things happening, just as my sister's childlike innocence was no warranty against cancer.

Those jolts were a sobering awareness that, no matter how hard you tried or how good people were, sad and bad things happened. It's not fair. Even the things that seemed fair, I wondered, were they truly fair? Or was it just luck? How much of what seems fair is actually about fairness after all? How much of it is about serendipity, how much is accident, how much is scientific bias? How much have we claimed to be as a result of our goodness or hard work when it was simply about timing?

I'm rubbing my temples as I write this, trying to pin it down. I want to pursue fairness in life, fairness in how I treat those I care about, fairness in my work. But I also accept that life isn't fair. A lot of it is outside of my awareness, it is a series of events, many of which I have no control over. I must pursue fairness in life while accepting that life itself isn't fair.

Why deny?

So, why is it so important for us to believe in fairness, to hold on to the idea that if we are good, kind and hardworking, then we will somehow protect ourselves from bad and sad things happening? Here are some ideas as to why you may struggle with facing the uncomfortable truth that life just isn't fair.

- **Because good things happen to good people** You see good things happening to good people. Those who work hard often get better results; those who invest in friendships kindly often have good people around them. Yes, being good often welcomes good, and so it is a drive to strive. You take inspiration from those who have achieved, you look for formulas and guidance and self-help in order to reach the goals others have mastered. Believing that good things happen to good people is motivating.

- **Unfairness is tough** The idea of fairness often evokes a feeling of safety. Maybe you have suffered somehow because you've been treated unfairly and so you pursue fairness with all of your might. You'll fight for fairness, you'll fight for other people, you'll fight until the right or fair thing happens because you've experienced how painful unfairness can be.

- **School teaches that hard work is rewarded** From early childhood, you are taught that if you work hard, you will be rewarded with a good job.

You are shown that you get out what you put in, as if life is all checks and balances and someone is keeping close, karmic tabs.

- **To try to avoid pain** You may try to avoid accepting the truth that life is unfair because you hope that fairness can protect you from pain and heartbreak. If you're good to someone, you hope they will be fair and be good to you. If you work hard at your job, you hope you won't lose it.

To recognize that life isn't fair brings us face to face with emotions like injustice, frustration, anger and grief. Those are justified feelings, it's just that they're not the nice, happy ones we often seek. But there is so much we can do with those feelings and I'm going to give you some ideas in a moment. First, we are going to look at the benefits of accepting the truth that life isn't fair.

The benefits of embracing this uncomfortable truth

Here are some of the benefits to enjoy when you begin to soften into the truth that life just isn't fair. See which ones resonate with you. Notice how much energy you consume fighting losing battles with other people in your life, and think about how much you'll gain when you begin to preserve that energy to use for other more fruitful purposes.

- **Stop fighting battles you're unlikely to win**
  You will be less likely to exhaust yourself trying to fight for fairness with those who have absolutely no interest in fairness. Perhaps you know someone who has a vested interest in things not being fair. Maybe they are making money through swindling the system or taking advantage of a partner's kindness. You want fairness but they don't. You see injustice and it makes your blood boil, but sometimes it feels like you're fighting a battle alone and it just works to make you angrier. You can choose to be honest with that person as to how you feel when you observe their behaviour or how it impacts you. And, if you choose, you can make yourself available should they want to talk about changing their ways. However, recognizing that you cannot change someone's mind if they aren't open to it will save you lots of energy-sapping frustration and anger.

- **Discover more resilience** When you begin to come to terms with the fact that, sometimes, life simply isn't fair, then you are less likely to find yourself stuck in the role of the 'victim'. When we see ourselves only as a victim of life's circumstances, it's hard to feel motivated and empowered to do what is within our control to move forward or change it. Accepting unfairness as a part of life enables you to feel more empowered rather than hopeless or helpless.

- **Feel motivated by unfairness rather than overwhelmed by it** When you find it hard to accept any unfairness, you may sometimes feel overwhelmed by feelings of injustice and frustration that things are the way they are and that circumstances may not change, or may be hard to change. However, a bit of acceptance for life's unfairness doesn't mean you'll become inactive, but you'll feel less hopeless and more empowered to fight for fairness, for change, and to advocate for others within the realm of your current resources and ability. It means that you'll be more likely to consider what you are able to and not able to do, rather than feeling stifled by the enormity of need.

Five ways to live with unfairness

People work hard and struggle financially. People are loved and not loved back. And yet we are taught that we can control things if we try hard enough. So, what can you do to feel a little bit more accepting of this truth? What can you do to help let go of some of the frustration that rises up around the things that you cannot control? How can you channel the rage that you feel when you witness something that just simply isn't fair?

1. Validate your emotions when you can't change the situation

When you feel like something is unfair and there's nothing you can actually do about it, make a choice to acknowledge and validate your feelings. Perhaps you've had a phone call with some sad news and you feel like life has dealt a cruel blow. Maybe you've missed out on a promotion to someone else who you truly believe is less qualified.

It can be tempting to swallow down the feelings or channel them into rage, but I recommend naming them as they move and shift. Sometimes we can worry that if we dwell on emotions, they linger for longer. Actually, the opposite is true. When we suppress, judge or try to manipulate emotions, they can come out sideways, perhaps in anger or irritability, and impact our behaviour and relationships.

One of my top tips is naming your feelings by way of validating them. It's a simple but effective way of giving them a voice and acknowledging them, which can sometimes be all we need in order to feel validated. Another way to validate your feelings is to speak about them with someone who cares, or try writing about them in a journal. Avoid the temptation to 'look on the bright side' and find your own grounding within it somehow.

For me, this can look like saying to myself: 'I'm feeling sad today, this doesn't feel fair.' Instead of trying to override the feelings with a positive mental attitude or beat myself up for lacking resilience, I am learning to notice my feelings and to trust that they change shape and intensity as I allow them to move through me.

My client Filippo found this small practice hugely helpful. Since he was a teenager he'd felt marginalized within his own family due to his sexuality. He had moved through a process of grieving that home no longer felt like a place to retreat to. Every time he visited his mother and brother, he tried so hard to help them understand him in the hope they might feel better able to accept him. However, regardless of how he articulated his story or tried to educate them, he'd leave feeling more acutely misunderstood and increasingly angry. This anger had begun to impact his sleep and his general feeling of well-being.

We identified another layer of grieving to be walked through: the grief that his mother and brother weren't willing to be open-minded and to truly know Filippo. It wasn't fair that he didn't feel accepted in his own family unit, as everyone deserves to feel loved and supported. Tapping into this sense of unfairness, and validating it, enabled my client to experience a powerful shift of acceptance. He discovered that as he became more accepting of the fact that his mother and brother weren't currently willing to 'see him' for who he was, he could channel the energy previously consumed by his anger into investing in relationships and friendships in which he felt supported and understood.

In acknowledging your feelings and letting them be as they are, you may recognize how quickly very active feelings of rage and frustration can move into feelings of sadness or helplessness.

It is also helpful to speak to those who understand how it feels to have to accept the uncomfortable truth of your specific situation. Just as my client found it helpful to voice his feelings of being marginalized with friends who understood, perhaps you can seek a support group online or offline who echo your feelings and validate them. Sometimes it means the world to hear someone say, 'Oh yes, I've been there, it's so tough, right?', or speak to someone who's a little further down the line in the journey for some hope and perspective.

2. Step out of victimhood

When we see ourselves as victims, our focus is on self-protection and nursing our wounds. We stop being proactive and it becomes harder to move through any pain or anger. In therapy, often people begin to get insights into how certain relationships in childhood impacted them. They make the connection that some of their present-day feelings, actions and behaviours are driven by historic hurts.

Over the years, I've had a number of clients pursue therapy sessions with me because they really want to settle down and consider having a family but their relationships don't seem to last the test of time. They've dated a lot but after a certain amount of time they feel increasingly uncomfortable, so they begin to disengage emotionally, which inevitably leads to the end of the relationship. My clients and I often identify that this make-or-break moment tends to happen when the mundanity of real life kicks in.

With my client Zeena, we concluded that once the honeymoon highs had passed, her relationships required a little more work, intentional connection and vulnerability in order to thrive. We identified that her father was emotionally withdrawn and would often mysteriously leave the home for a period of time, not saying when he'd be back. We recognized that she felt unsafe in relationships as soon as they got serious, partly because she subconsciously feared that the other person would leave and partly because she didn't have enough of a sense of safety and consistency in childhood to learn that she could be vulnerable and open, and people wouldn't run away. As a child, Zeena believed it was her fault that her father kept leaving.

As we talked about this, Zeena felt so angry. 'How dare my father do this to me as a kid? How dare my father mess me so much so that I can't find love for myself? I have been robbed, I will never settle down, I will never know what it feels like to be safe. My father could have had a loving family but he threw it away, and now he's stopped me from having one too.'

Can you imagine what would happen if the process ended there and Zeena stayed stuck in the recognition that she was a victim and that her father hadn't modelled security as he ideally should have? She would live with so much anger and pain. She believed she had been robbed of her 'right'. Nursing the anger and believing that her future had been broken by the story of her past would ironically make it less likely for her to find what she yearned for.

Fortunately, you can be a victim and decide not to lean into victimhood. Or you can recognize where you've lived feeling like the victim and you now want to move forward. To do this, you must have your feelings heard and validated. My client had to step out of victimhood to learn to take small risks of vulnerability. Then she would slowly learn to have deep and healthy connections. Her father left her, but not everyone would. Life isn't fair. Her father's own childhood story would likely explain why he was the way he was. Whether my client would ever hear that story or not didn't mean she couldn't pursue a different story for herself.

So choose to let go of any victim mentality that is keeping you stuck. Victim mentality is that feeling that the world is against you. Perhaps someone hurt you and you didn't deserve it. Yes, it was bad, so allow yourself to dwell on that for a bit. But don't get stuck there for too long. Consider how you can act so that you can feel empowered again to reclaim your story and your future as your own.

A good way to act upon this is to answer these questions:

- *Where am I struggling with unfairness in my life?*
- *What feelings do I experience? What is the cost of holding on to this unfairness?*
- *If I begin to accept this unfairness, where else might I direct that energy? What other relationships in which I enjoy feeling understood and supported might benefit from this time and energy instead?*

As you work through this exercise, identify where you might need therapeutic support in this, just to untangle it a little bit.

3. Let yourself grieve the lack of fairness

As the truth that life isn't fair really settles in, allow yourself to grieve the idea of fairness if you need to. It's sad that some things just aren't fair. I have walked beside a friend of mine through her multiple baby losses, one of which happened almost at the same time as I welcomed my own healthy baby. How come I had three living babies and she had none? It wasn't fair. Oh, how I wished it was fair.

A client's story echoed my own. She came to speak to me as her treasured relationship with her sister felt strained and uncomfortable for 'the first time in my life'. Her sister had just experienced a failed round of IVF after trying to start a family for five years. My client, Jenna, who had two young children, had begun to struggle with feelings of guilt and had been finding it hard to be normal around her sister: 'I just feel so bad. I'd placed all my hope in the fact the IVF would work for her, and that the guilt would ease. She really needs me now, but I just feel so aware that I have what she wants.'

We identified those feelings of unfairness. It didn't feel fair that Jenna had her children and her sister didn't. Her deep desire for things to feel 'fair' meant that she was finding it hard to not only talk to her sister, but to enjoy her own family: 'Every time I look at my kids, I feel overwhelmed by my sister's struggle. I feel bad for enjoying them.'

143

In our sessions, Jenna allowed herself to grapple with the lack of fairness and find ways to articulate it to her sister. She began to feel a confidence in talking to her again: 'Instead of avoiding talking about my kids, I could talk about how I felt about the fact that [she and her husband] were going through such a hard time, and how I was grieving with her. My sister opened up about her feelings of jealousy and said it felt like a relief to be able to voice them rather than to pressure herself to push them down. Approaching it like this helped me be more present with my own kids as I could accept both the good in my life and my feelings of sadness for my sister.' This guilt could have stopped Jenna from enjoying what was in front of her, and perhaps in time it might have further fractured her relationship with her sister.

Maybe, like Jenna, you might consider how in your life you need to grieve a lack of fairness rather than keep fighting it. Take a moment to write down some of the wider feelings around an unfairness that you face. Maybe you feel nudged to talk about this with someone so that you can meet them more authentically as you choose to remove an elephant from the corner of the room!

Finding a more peaceful acceptance of the truth that life isn't fair requires us to let go of entitlement. Entitlement is the belief that life treats us as we deserve: 'If I want kids, I'm entitled to kids. If I want a job, life should give me a job.' It's good to go after good things that we want, but life promises nothing. It's not equal. Criminals can live to the ripe old age of ninety and life's saints can die young. I was never owed or promised three healthy kids by the world. I am not entitled to happiness, a job, security, love. Just as my friend wasn't owed loss.

So, let go of the belief that everyone is entitled to great things. It's humbling to realize how much in your life came to you because of luck, or timing, or the chance meeting of healthy sperm with healthy egg. It's a sobering realization but it nudges you towards awareness of your privilege and a sense of gratitude. You might have worked hard to increase the chances of good things happening but life doesn't owe you anything because it's not fair like that. You cannot control the outcome as much as you think.

This isn't doom and gloom. If you think about it, it's actually really liberating. If what happens isn't fundamentally and entirely a result of your input, then you can let go of some of the anger or injustice you feel. Also, you can enjoy good things coming your way that you've never earned or deserved. Sometimes your good works won't be rewarded. Recognize them. Write them down. Choose to allow yourself to be proud and clap for yourself even if nobody else will. Just because your goodness isn't recognized, it doesn't mean you didn't do well.

Life isn't fair and sometimes you may receive less – or even far more – than you believe you deserve. I spent too long feeling undeserving of the wonderful people in my life, but I've come to realize that it's not about my deserving, because I was never entitled to it. I wasn't owed it, it's just a blessing, and I recognize it as a privilege. I feel a sense of calm as I consider that I don't have to make sense of it all, I just have to accept it and grieve it where needed. Grief makes way for gentle acceptance, after all.

4. Find your fight

Rage is an energizing feeling, isn't it? Consider how it feels in your body. I experience it as a hot emotion, one that drives me to do something, be it shout, throw, fight or run. Rage activates your nervous system stress response because something has triggered a feeling of threat. A sense of unfairness can feel threatening to your safety. As you become more accepting of life's unfairness, this may well soften.

However, sometimes it's good to allow the rage to move you to action. Rage that stems from injustice can prompt change in the world. Every charity, every changed law, every campaign to see fairness for a people, group or marginalized community most likely began with rage. While sometimes in life we'd do better to step back from a fight against unfairness and just accept it, at other times we might feel like the situation calls us to step towards the fight instead.

During the pandemic I felt a simmering sense of injustice at how many new mothers missed out on emotional support due to the lockdowns. The red-hot, passion-filled emotion fuelled me to do a free online series of talks to educate and support new mothers in the things I felt they needed to know, in order to improve their emotional well-being and lessen the likelihood of postnatal anxiety and depression. The recognition of how unfair this felt meant that over 10,000 women benefited from my four free sessions, and the feedback confirmed that it had been the right thing to do. I acted off the back of an injustice and something good came of it.

In a similar way, one of my clients, after returning to his desk post-pandemic lockdowns, felt angered by the immediate resorting to presenteeism. He spoke to numerous colleagues only to discover that they too felt more trusted and much happier with the autonomy that the forced working from home had brought. During the lockdown, Kevin, my client, had been fulfilling his workload as normal, but had benefited from the opportunity to do a workout before lunch or to walk the dog during daylight hours.

In the office, the culture had been that 'if you weren't at your desk, it was assumed you wouldn't get the work done'. Kevin and a couple of colleagues spoke to numerous friends and contacts about their own work cultures, many of which were more flexible and accommodating of amended working hours. It didn't feel fair. They called a meeting to ask to trial a more flexible working environment. After three months, it was agreed that the health, happiness and, much to the board's surprise, output of the workforce had increased. Thus the more flexible approach became permanent, all thanks to Kevin's frustration!

Leaning into your sense of injustice can lead you to change circumstances, outlooks, laws and lives. If there's a specific injustice that continues to make you angry, consider how you might channel that rage to fight for change. Write it down in your journal and ask yourself how you could harness some of that rageful or frustrated energy and turn it into action. If you can't join a community or group that reflects your passion and invites you to join the fight then create one. The internet is amazing for this! Whether your righteous anger is for animal rights, political shifts, saving the planet or an end to child slavery, join forces with others or pledge to support a charity somehow. It feels great to channel your anger in a way that is productive.

When we channel our rage, it saves it from spurting out unhelpfully. I had a friend who was so angry about the impact that idling cars had on the environment that she'd be seething in her car every time she saw someone pause with their engine on. It impacted her relationships as much as her blood pressure. She joined an online community who channelled their righteous anger into creating warm, approachable information and posters that educated people on why they should switch their engines off when they stopped their cars for any length of time. The knowledge that she was working on the bigger picture of educating people meant that her anger was less directed at specific individuals.

5. Be fair where you can

Choose to be fair, where you can. Sometimes you do have control over whether you can make a fair decision or not. Isn't choosing fairness often the same as choosing kindness? Isn't it also often synonymous with being authentic? Kindness, authenticity and fairness are brilliant qualities, and we become those things through the words we speak and the things we do.

This isn't true all of the time, of course. Sometimes the thing that is fair isn't received well by the other person. Or in speaking out your authentic truth and setting a boundary, another person might feel a sense of frustration and injustice because they've benefited from your lack of boundaries in the past!

My client sought sessions with me after going on holiday with his partner. They had spent a week abroad with another couple and it had been eye-opening for Jon. 'The way they spoke to each other was so different to how my wife and I communicated. They were kinder, and didn't put each other down at all. Obviously, they were likely on good behaviour as we were around, but their whole relationship just seemed healthier and happier and I realized quite how mean to each other we were.'

Over the following months, Jon spoke in depth about the dynamics in his relationship, and how at times he and his wife were hurting each other through their words and actions. Jon shared how unhappy he had felt, and how witnessing another couple had shone a light on their dysfunction. He regularly asked his wife to undergo couples therapy with him, in order to find ways to restore some gentleness and kindness into their relationship, but she would receive the suggestion as an attack and the dynamic would intensify. Over the coming months, Jon spiralled into a deeper sense of disconnection and hurt, and the relationship ended. He felt devastated that she hadn't been able to commit, alongside him, to working on the harmful dynamics they shared.

So, yes, it's important to acknowledge that sometimes someone isn't able to honour a request for fairness or kindness, or a circumstance cannot be changed through your own strength alone. That can be hard and painful, and sometimes even lead to the fracturing of a relationship and subsequent grief.

As you move through your week, begin to notice the opportunities that arise to act fairly. Perhaps a friend or colleague gets given an opportunity that you wanted. Notice any sense of entitlement that bubbles up in you: 'That's not fair, I wanted that, I should have been given it.' Your inner child might want to sabotage it for the other person somehow, maybe by speaking critically of the opportunity in order to make it less attractive for the both of you.

As you reflect on these moments, write them down and consider how you can make the choice to validate your authentic emotions so that they don't spurt out sideways, while also accepting the uncomfortable truth that life isn't fair. Perhaps you respond to your colleague by saying, 'Wow, that's amazing. If I'm honest, I feel a bit envious as I'd love that opportunity, but I can't wait to hear how you get on. Enjoy it!'

We can choose to be unfair; we can go after something we know someone else deserves; we can hurt someone to protect our own sense of self and ego. Try not to compare your situation or your opportunities with what you see of others because it's not all checks and balances and it doesn't all add up.

Conclusion

So, you have faced the uncomfortable truth that life isn't fair and perhaps it's beginning to feel less rage-inducing than it did before you turned to this chapter. But don't forget that just because life often isn't fair, it's dangerous to lie back and let the unfairness roll over us. Seeking fairness where we can means there will be more justice and equality in our societies.

Accepting that life isn't always fair prevents you from holding on to anger for longer than you need to. It paves the way for healthy grief, which may feel sad and tough, but to allow yourself to grieve is so important. Grieve the times you feel hard done by, badly treated or when unfairness has meant you've missed out or lost. Grieve what was robbed from you, the loss of a hope or a dream, or an opportunity that was swept out of sight by someone else. Grief makes way for gentle, soothing acceptance.

As you pursue fairness, you will navigate some difficult conversations, you will place new boundaries and you may find yourself speaking up for yourself and others. But not only this, you will also nurture self-respect, which in turn helps grow confidence and self-esteem.

JOURNAL POINTS

1. What in your life has felt unfair? Have you allowed yourself to grieve that?
2. What have you felt entitled to?
3. If you feel rage against an injustice, what move can you make to channel this productively?

Life isn't fair, but I'll seek fairness anyway

6.

I am Not Good Enough

Diving headfirst into the uncomfortable truth

You're not good enough.

Well, this really contrasts with the positive mantras printed on T-shirts and the cursive affirmations that skip across your social media feeds, doesn't it?

Whether you have positive affirmations on every mirror in your house or not, you may find that no matter how many times you repeat them to yourself, they just don't seem to shift the constant feeling that you're not good enough. Not good enough for who? Not good enough for what? You want to get away from this feeling. You want to believe that 'You're enough', just like the words proclaim.

I'm here to tell you that one of the main reasons you don't feel good enough is because you're not. You're not good enough. You, with your limited resources of time, energy and patience, and your human body that gets sick and tired, you who responds to the world with emotions, and sometimes makes decisions based on narratives and beliefs that are set so deeply in your brain that you don't even realize you're dancing to their beats. You with the toxic traits no matter how many self-help books you inhale. You with the vulnerable and breakable heart.

You are never going to be enough for what the world and some of the people around you want you to be. You're never going to be enough for some of the standards set for you by yourself and others.

When you begin to accept the uncomfortable truth that you are not enough, you can start to find more respect for your boundaries and the limits of your resources rather than asking yourself to plough through them.

Good enough for what? Good enough for who?

As you move through this chapter, I want to clarify what I mean by 'you're not good enough'. I believe there are two types of 'not good enough', and here they are:

First, you've got the not-good-enoughness that comes from a feeling of shame and 'wrongness'. You don't feel like you're good enough for good things. This is fundamentally untrue, and this narrative has come from the way in which you've been treated and spoken to, or the way you've had to internalize feelings because you felt that you weren't accepted or loved by caregivers when you responded or behaved a certain way. Instead of someone helping you process the difficulty, you were led to believe that *you* were the difficulty.

Dev, one of my clients, shared something that encapsulates this brilliantly: 'My family moved from Delhi to Wales when I was six. I felt different to everyone around me. My teachers shortened my name in order to make it easier to pronounce, and my friends at school would mimic my accent and laugh at my lunch. I tried to change as quickly as I could, to blend in, to feel accepted. I grew up feeling I had to hide my true self as if there was something unacceptable about it. I felt like an imposter in my own life.' Dev hadn't done anything 'wrong' and yet he had internalized this feeling of not-good-enoughness due to the way he had been treated.

The second feeling of 'not good enough' comes when you expect yourself to be able to do more than you humanly can. You are unlikely to feel 'good enough' when you struggle to accept your limited resources and your messy, imperfect humanness. Or you find it hard to find peace with the fact that you don't have enough knowledge to get everything right, you don't have enough energy to be all things to all people, you don't have enough time to get everything on your list done. You don't have enough insight to say the right things to everyone all the time. You don't have enough physical or mental strength to carry the weight of everyone's expectations.

Kelly shared in one of our sessions how she was the 'office "yes" woman'. She'd hide her frustration, resentment and exhaustion and show willing to take on any role or project asked of her. 'It was only when my colleague went off on long-term sick leave that I broke. It was expected that I'd carry her workload, but it was too much.' In time, Kelly felt able to tell her boss that she didn't have the capacity to carry out the enormous workload and gave a small insight into the struggle she'd been having behind the scenes.

Together, we identified that Kelly had gained a sense of purpose through accepting extra work, yet hadn't been acknowledging or respecting her own limits. Her boss agreed to find temporary support to help ease the workload and Kelly literally felt a weight lifted from her shoulders. 'I began to start enjoying work again, and will always make sure I take into account what is already on my plate before I consider adding to it.'

So, as you move through this chapter, keep these two forms of not-good-enoughness in mind as we challenge and unpick this truth. My hope is that, as you reflect, you'll begin to welcome the uncomfortable truth of your not-good-enoughness with open arms, just as Kelly did.

My story

For the majority of my life I've believed that I wasn't enough. Enough for what, you ask? I didn't believe I was good enough to be loved, I didn't feel I was acceptable or fun enough to be befriended. I didn't think I was worthy enough to be loved by my kids. I didn't believe I was clever enough to thrive in a job I loved. So, I tried hard at everything. I aimed high. And it worked: I had friends, I had loving kids and a good job. I was loved and accepted.

However, I felt like I was an imposter in my own life. David Smail, in his book *Illusion and Reality: The Meaning of Anxiety*, encapsulates how I felt. He says:

> Much of our waking life is spent in a desperate struggle to persuade others that we are not what we fear ourselves to be, or what they may discover us to be if they see through our pretences. Most people, most of the time, have a profound and unhappy awareness of the contrast between what they are and what they ought to be.

Because of this distance between how I portrayed myself and how I truly was, I believed I was only deemed good enough by others because I was trying so hard. I truly felt that if people knew how much I really resented some of the things I agreed to do, when in fact I had little capacity to give out, they'd be shocked. If people knew how much of my opinion I was swallowing down out of fear of offending them, or how many of my needs I wasn't voicing in order to avoid burdening them, then they'd change their minds about me. They'd realize that I wasn't worthy of their time, energy, love and acceptance after all.

I believe this came about due to childhood trauma. When we're little, we're egocentric. That means we believe everything is about us. Therefore if someone isn't able to give you a sense of unconditional acceptance, you come to the conclusion that it's because you aren't enough somehow.

And what do we do when we don't feel enough for a caregiver? As a child, you are vulnerable, you need your caregiver for safety, you need to do what you can for them to be on your side in order for you to survive. So, you try to be good, you try to compensate; you might push down emotions that seem to push them away.

I went through a lot of my life believing that I was only acceptable if and because I was good and giving and loving and sacrificial, and I'd say 'yes' regardless of the cost. And then I became a mother and suddenly there was a whole new role in which I needed to prove my enoughness. During a painfully difficult period of mothering, in which I had tried so hard to fly the flag of

'I've got this', it became too much. The expectations I'd placed upon myself were too much, too high, too hard.

One day, as friends staged an intervention and told me that they knew I wasn't okay, I had to come face to face with the truth of my not-enoughness. I needed to take a different tack. I had to acknowledge that I needed people. I felt everything in me exhale when I began to accept that I was never going to be good enough to keep everyone happy, to achieve everything I wanted, to do everything to perfection. I began to work with my limits rather than see them as weaknesses. I began to seek and accept support because I recognized that I wasn't enough to do everything on my own.

Raising the white flag of surrender to seeking and earning, driving and striving to find a sense of my enoughness, was one of the best things I ever did. Yes, I am strong and capable, and I am also vulnerable and limited and needing. Not because I'm weak, but because I'm human.

Why deny?

As you've read through my own reasons for denying my not-good-enoughness, I wonder if any of them resonated with you? Have a look at the following reasons as to why you might have been sidestepping the liberating truth that you're not good enough.

- **Media's portrayal of humanness** Media feeds us so many different filtered versions of reality. As humans, we are hardwired to believe what we see. Think about magic tricks. Cognitively we know it's a trick of the hand or eye, but it still feels so confusing and surprising. In the same way, media creates a Frankenstein of perfection which intellectually we know doesn't exist, but when it's coming at us from all angles, it's tough not to start believing it.

- **Increased juggle without increased energy and time** The demands on your time are higher than ever, yet you still have the same hours in the day. Consider the things that fight for your attention now that wouldn't have been the same for the previous generation. The nine-to-five doesn't really exist any more and there are always notifications flashing somewhere. The number of calls on your attention is higher than ever, yet you don't have any more hours in the day or any more energy to navigate them. You're fighting today's demands under yesterday's standards.

- **We are sold more** There is always more you can be and there are ways to become faster, more efficient. You'll find endless life hacks, tips and tricks that help squeeze everything out of your resources. Marketing reminds you that you're lacking somehow, before it swiftly swoops in and suggests the answer. If you truly came to terms with the fact that you'll never be 'enough' by the world's standards, then imagine how much money you'd save!

- **You have critical inner chatter** If you have a cruel or bullying inner critic, then you're likely to struggle with believing that you are likeable, loveable and acceptable. If you treat an animal unkindly for long enough, they will fail to feel safe with anyone. In the same way, if your internal chatter is largely impatient or critical, then it can feel tough to receive kind words and actions from others.

- **You didn't receive unconditional acceptance in childhood or you've been through trauma** Before I elaborate on this thought, I have noticed that 'trauma' is a term that is used increasingly widely and colloquially in our culture, sometimes flippantly: 'Oh, that was a traumatic trip into the office.' I'd like to clarify that trauma in its true sense is an emotional response to a scenario in which someone was, or felt, acutely or dangerously unsafe, be it physically or mentally. Someone may experience trauma if they feel physically or psychologically overwhelmed or threatened, either in a shocking situation in which they felt out of control or through feeling chronically unsafe in a relationship or circumstance. Trauma can trigger a range of physical and mental symptoms such as shock, disconnection, upset and anxiety. When a person experiences trauma, it can also lead to post-traumatic stress disorder (PTSD), which impacts day-to-day well-being and benefits from psychological support and tools to help regain a sense of calm and safety.

So, with that in mind, be aware that experiencing trauma in childhood which isn't processed or therapeutically addressed can feed into a sense of not being good enough. Perhaps an adult or caregiver was chronically unavailable either physically (to meet needs and comfort) or emotionally (to help you navigate emotion and provide a secure and loving space for you). Maybe there was a particular traumatic event that overshadowed the typical play, ease and fun of childhood. Perhaps you sensed or learned that people couldn't be trusted to meet your needs so you needed to meet them alone. You've internalized the idea that you have to be strong and self-sufficient and that to need people is a failure or a weakness. To not feel good enough feels like a shameful thing, so you must earn your acceptance.

Heavy stuff, hey? I really just want to come in here with a huge promise of hope. Just as internal dialogues are learned and rehearsed over years, they can be relearned. Just as our subconscious narrative has been fed by the media's call of 'you need to be more', we can become aware of it so we can recognize the choices that we do actually have. Just as people have shaped our broken beliefs that to not be good enough is somehow failure, we can learn to grow in confidence by placing fresh boundaries and allowing people to support us.

So, before you find out how on earth you get to this place, let's highlight the benefits of accepting the uncomfortable truth that you'll never be enough, and that it's not a bad thing!

The benefits of embracing this uncomfortable truth

In slowly embracing the uncomfortable truth that you won't always be good enough, you'll feel less duped by the external narratives you see around you, and you'll find more acceptance of your imperfect humanness. As you find ways to be more open with others about your limits and shortfalls, you'll discover fresh energy gained from a decreased need to people-please. So, take some time to acquaint yourself with the following benefits to welcoming a new appreciation of not-good-enoughness.

- **You'll welcome more rest** The less you strive to feel like you're good enough, the more you recognize the little and not-so-little signals that your body gives you in order to tell you to slow down. You'll be more likely to accept what opportunities for rest arise, rather than shutting them down with relentless 'doing', or drowning them out with pep talks to 'try harder'. You'll lessen the likelihood of the burnout that happens when you repeatedly push beyond the limits of your resources.

- **Stop people-pleasing** Imagine you've made a big chocolate cake covered in thick buttercream. You know people like cake, so you give wedges away freely in return for the look of enjoyment on their faces. When you feel a swell of hunger rise up, you look down at the plate in anticipation. You see crumbs. When you step out of the cycle of engaging in people-pleasing behaviour, you can choose to be more intentional about where you invest your time and energy. This means you'll be far less likely to feel like you're left with a plate of crumbs. Instead, you'll have some time and energy left at the end of the day so you won't feel frazzled and resentful. Boundaries become clearer and you'll find a little more breathing space in your mind and diary.

- **Stronger self-esteem** If your fundamental sense of not being good enough is rooted in low self-esteem rather than an acceptance of your limited resources, you may feel like you're a problem you need to fix. However, when you accept that you're flawed and you're just trying your best with the knowledge and resources you have, you're less likely to beat yourself up for the times you inevitably get things wrong. You'll recognize that growth is a bumpy upwards trajectory rather than a need to get it right all the time.

- **Feel more authentic** When you compensate your internal feeling of not-good-enoughness with trying to prove yourself externally in the things you do and say, then you might feel like an imposter. But as you embrace the different layers of yourself, and how they can all exist within the whole – the capable, the insecure, the confident, the anxious – then the sense of imposter syndrome will ebb away. Whether it's at work or in your friendships, the more you acknowledge your human, limited, messy, vulnerable self, the less exhausted you'll feel by holding up that false facade. As you find the confidence to be more open and honest in your meaningful relationships, that sense of 'if they really knew me, they wouldn't like me' will also fade away.

- **Experience more of what life has to offer** If your feeling of not-good-enoughness is rooted in shame then you may feel undeserving of good things. But as you embrace your own limits and humanness, that sense of valuing yourself will bring fresh confidence and a sense of deservedness in seeking new experiences and pushing your own boundaries. You will find yourself pondering whether you should throw caution to the wind and apply for that job, or try that new hobby even though you'll probably be a little bad at it to begin with.

I wonder what else you've dreamed about as you've read these benefits. Make a note of any new realizations you've had as writing them down helps them become more conscious.

Five ways to accept your limitations

How can you become more accepting of the truth that you're never going to be enough for the standards placed upon you by yourself and the world, so that you can live within your means? Here are five ways to help you live out this uncomfortable, liberating truth.

1. Question the 'should's

Think of how often you feel like you 'should' do a particular thing or feel a particular way. 'Should's are like little rules that you live by, which shape and dictate the decisions you make and how you portray and express yourself. Consider some of the 'should's you've uttered to yourself today: *I should have worked harder at that project; I should work out today; I shouldn't have felt upset about that; I should definitely go for those social drinks tonight even though I'm exhausted.*

Ask yourself what 'should's you might need to challenge. *I should be able to please everyone, I should always be calm, I should always get things right on the first try.* Are these 'should's realistic? Are they inspired by perfectionism and people-pleasing or are they driven by shame and guilt? Is your self-esteem and confidence hinging on the outcome?

Recognizing what is driving that feeling gives you a choice of whether to lean into it or to challenge it. When you find yourself thinking you 'should' do, choose or feel a particular thing, follow it with the question 'Should I?' Consider what your gut might be saying.

This has been a game-changer for me and is something that I often challenge clients with too. Every time I hear a 'should' pop up, I enquire as to the rule that is being followed. Who set the rule and is it right for you to keep it?

As I write, I recall one client who had believed she shouldn't go travelling as a teenager because she was concerned that her mother would 'worry too much'. She told me: 'I know it was ten years ago, but that was my chance. I saw how my mum struggled with me going to college, so I thought I shouldn't take a gap year as the idea of her worrying constantly felt awful. I didn't want to do that to her.' Ten years down the line, her relationship with her mother had become fractured by her mum's controlling behaviour and her inability to respect my client's desire to accept a job in a neighbouring city. As she reflected on how many other things she hadn't experienced because she felt she 'shouldn't rock the boat for Mum', she began to experience a mixture of grief and resentment at how her mother's unaddressed anxiety had limited her.

One day she came into our session and declared that she had asked her boss for a sabbatical and was planning on taking some time out to travel. I delighted in seeing her enjoy challenging the 'should's in different areas of her life, and watching her grow in confidence as she did so.

I remember when I decided to stop sending Christmas cards. It was one admin job too many. 'I should send Christmas cards,' I thought. 'It's what my mother does, it's what I've always done.' Resenting the job of buying cards and stamps before I'd even begun it, I asked myself 'Should I?' I recognized that nobody was making me. Sure, someone might wonder where our annual card was, but if anyone judged me, I knew my truth, and the truth was that I didn't have capacity to do it all so something had to go. Question your 'should's too and you'll begin to see that many of them are actually up for negotiation.

2. Try the litmus test

Frank sat in my therapy room trying to untangle his feelings of not being good enough in his new relationship. He was so happy with his new partner and they'd 'fallen in love in a whirlwind' after meeting on a dating app: 'It was love at first sight. Like in the movies. We moved in together within a month! I know it sounds ridiculous. She's amazing and I'm just always feeling like it's too good to be true and that she'll suddenly look at me and regret being with me.' Frank felt that his feeling of not being good enough for his new partner was impacting his behaviour. He was exhausting himself trying to get 'everything right' and was at times anxious and losing sleep due to ruminating over things he may have done to 'burst the bubble'.

I invited Frank to use my 'litmus test' against his feelings of not being good enough to provide him with some clarity. We worked through these questions together:

- *Is my feeling of not-good-enoughness fuelling people-pleasing or perfectionist behaviour?*
- *In my assessment of myself, how much am I taking into account my messy humanness?*
- *Where am I looking for reassurance? How sustainable is this source of reassurance and*

*self-esteem? What is the cost and risk of seeking my
reassurance here?*

- *How might I seek more sustainable reassurance? What
  might need to be challenged or changed regarding my
  perception of myself, my boundaries, my expectations
  or my circumstances?*

This helped Frank determine that his feelings of not-good-
enoughness were causing his behaviour towards his
partner to be driven by fear. He reflected that he wasn't
taking into account his humanness and was seeking to
portray himself as a 'perfect partner'. He sought
reassurance in her response to his gestures and
behaviour: 'I wanted to see that she was happy with me, all
the time. It must be a bit exhausting, come to think of it.'
He recognized that the cost of seeking reassurance from
his partner that he *was* good enough was probably fuelling
his sleepless nights as she wouldn't always be able to give
it to him as often as he felt he needed it.

In the following sessions, Frank and I worked on ways to
nurture his self-esteem and his acceptance of his naturally
imperfect nature. He had some light-bulb moments about
his childhood and, off the back of them, he had some really
honest, vulnerable conversations with his partner about both

of their childhoods. In time, he began to feel more at ease in the relationship and became more aware that both he and his partner brought with them a wealth of experiences, histories and personality traits. They learned to find new ways to communicate their needs and feelings.

Next time you don't feel good enough, move through these same litmus test questions. See what comes up and consider how perhaps the issue isn't that you're not good enough, but that you're expecting to be far better than you can humanly be.

3. Seek support and take steps in vulnerability

You are hardwired to need community, and the people around you have strengths in the same places you have weaknesses. Think about the Stone Age. Some early humans were physically more suited to hunting while others were better placed in the role of gathering or stoking the fire. Each role was vital for survival. We cannot all be good at everything, strong in every way and capable at everything we turn our hands to.

The less you try to be everything, the more you are able to let others step in with their skills so that you can focus on the things that play to your strengths.

By her own admission, Taya came to see me for therapy begrudgingly. 'I really felt that I should be able to make sense of my anxiety. I'm a clever woman. I'm a scientist! I know myself.' She saw therapy as a last-ditch attempt and felt a great sense of failure for not having been able to 'sort it out myself'. As we moved through subsequent sessions, Taya marvelled at the fact that she was learning new things about herself. We discussed how beneficial it is to get fresh eyes on a situation sometimes. She realized that seeking therapy wasn't admitting failure, but an opportunity to welcome someone else's valuable perspective. 'I guess nobody can see everything from every angle themselves,' she mused. This reflection was such a powerful reinforcement of what can happen when we welcome others in on our challenges.

I remember moving a large piece of furniture upstairs on my own. I did it out of impatience. I didn't want to wait for my partner to help me do it, and I wanted to show myself that I was strong enough. It was tough. I sweated, I pulled a muscle, I scratched the paint up the stairs, but I did it. I did it myself to prove that I could, but it came at a cost. It would have been better to recognize that it was a two-person job and wait. That wouldn't have been weakness, it would have been sensible.

You need people. It doesn't make you needy to need people, it's just an acknowledgement that you're not superhuman. Sure, someone might not be able to fix your situation, or remove your heartache, but they can walk alongside you as you trudge through that fire. Perhaps someone doesn't have the perfect words of wisdom to help you with your problem, but they might be able to offer you their own interpretation or perspective which brings a new route of thought for you.

I'd love you to consider this as you read. What needs do you have at the moment? Where might you have been trying to meet these needs alone when, in truth, you'd benefit from asking someone to walk alongside you or to offer a helping hand? Notice where it would do you good to realize that you're not good enough and begin to think of ways you might benefit from the support and insight of other people. Take small risks of vulnerability, begin to speak out your needs and feelings, and see how people respond. Sure, not everyone will 'get you' or have the capacity to be what you need, but that doesn't mean that nobody will.

4. Know the limits of your resources

My client Dan began our session yawning. He had got up
at four a.m. that morning to pick a friend up from the
airport in order to help him out. As we had been exploring
his tendency to lean into people-pleasing behaviours, I
asked him whether he had done it out of a drive to please
in order to feel deserving of the friendship, or as an act of
choice regardless of what gratitude he might receive.
'Well, when he asked me, I actually took a moment to think.
Usually I'd just say "yes" automatically, but this time I didn't
reply to his text immediately.' Dan thought about his day at
work and what time he might finish. He had no late
meetings. He asked himself if he wanted to invest in his
friend in this way, and whether he'd be hiding any
resentment at getting up at such an early hour that would
taint his kind gesture. He concluded that he would get an
early night and pick his friend up. I loved hearing Dan talk
through this process. It only took a moment for him, but
meant that his 'yes' was intentional and considered, and
therefore more authentic. Sometimes there can be a
sacrificial element to our relationships, but it is done
through choice rather than fear.

When I was training as a psychotherapist, I worked part-
time as a PA in a lovely marketing agency. To earn extra

money to pay my fees, I also did some simple training in gel manicures and I'd ride my bike around South London and sit in the corner of people's living rooms doing manicures as groups of women caught up and partied.

For a long time, whenever a friend came to visit, I'd insist on doing her nails or giving a massage regardless of how much energy or time I had to spare. This wasn't a simple kindly gesture but was rooted in a need to earn their friendship. I didn't believe that in and of myself I was worthy of their kindness, so I had to do something extra in order to feel close to deserving of their time.

So, as a takeaway, next time someone asks something of you, whether it be in a work or a social context, don't say a knee-jerk 'yes'. Adopt a pause. Let them know that you'll check your diary (even if you don't). This gives you an opportunity to consider what resources you have available to give, or whether you'll be putting yourself in the overdraft of your energy, money or time by saying 'yes'. When you say 'yes' wholeheartedly and authentically, it's a gift to the other person. When you say 'yes' but you're resentful and shouldering a big secret cost, you might get the job done, but repeatedly doing this will impact the relationship in time. When you neglect to assert healthy boundaries around your resources and energy, you can end up feeling used and taken for granted. There are many creative ways to say 'no', but being authentic in your response nurtures and honours your relationships, and yourself.

5. Question comparison

Everyone compares themselves to others, it's an inbuilt mechanism that drives us to conform and belong in order to secure our safety. We humans are pack animals. There is safety in numbers, and when you are accepted as part of a group or culture it is more likely that others will support and protect you if needs be. Comparing yourself to others means that you'll tend to gravitate towards those who you don't feel threatened by, or those who portray similarities to you, meaning that you're more likely to be accepted into 'the pack'.

But when comparison moves beyond 'That person has a better job than I do' and turns into 'I'm failing, I should be doing better, I'm not enough', then it begins to chip away at your confidence and sense of identity.

When you compare yourself to someone, you are dehumanizing yourself and the other person. Huh? That sounds a little harsh, right? Let me explain. When you compare someone's front-of-house to your behind-the-scenes reality, you are taking one part of their story, personality or outward achievement and using it as a bar to measure yourself against. You're overlooking the fact that they are a whole person. You're distilling them down to the one factor you see and you're drawing a conclusion about them.

I find that I often do this in terms of parenting. I see one mother being particularly calm with her kids, and I think, 'Wow, I'm such a rubbish parent.' I'm measuring a huge part of me against one tiny snapshot of her. How is this fair?

When you compare yourself in some way, you end up concluding that you're better or worse than the other person. You'll probably find that this temporarily boosts or knocks your self-esteem. If you look to everyone else to tell you whether you're good or not, your self-esteem will be sat firmly on that roller coaster, dipping and diving in response to whatever conclusion you've drawn.

My client Sofia spent a session reflecting on her childhood: 'At school, I just morphed into whoever I thought people wanted me to be. I would move around schools as my parents were in the army, and I'd be faced with a new school every couple of years. I'd literally stand alone in the lunch queue, look at the tables of people, think who I most looked like and try to mimic their likes and dislikes. Anything to fit in and feel accepted.' While Sofia told me that this actually tended to work, she was left feeling unsure of who she truly was. She felt exhausted going into new environments as she'd find herself cruelly comparing herself to others and constantly looking for cues and clues as to whether she was liked in an attempt to work out where she'd feel most safe and accepted.

If, like Sofia, comparison has become a habit for you, then here is a wonderful way to start to break out of the comparison habit. Next time you notice you're comparing yourself, be inquisitive. Turn the subjective 'He's better than me' into the factual 'I am watching him do the presentation in a more articulate way than I would be able to.' Then ask yourself 'What else is behind this comparison?' Perhaps it's envy, maybe you feel jealous, but instead of just criticizing yourself, you seek to brush up on your skills so that next time you present, you might do so more confidently. Perhaps you feel fearful of rejection, in which case you may benefit from investing in being more open and honest in some of those meaningful relationships that you have, in order to cultivate a sense of grounded acceptance.

Conclusion

Being authentic is the key to feeling empowered by the truth that you aren't enough. Recognize the needs, feelings and opinions that arise within you and choose to turn towards them and respect them, rather than always choosing to push through them, deny or squash them with criticism. In this way you'll grow to respect your limitations and boundaries rather than experiencing them as failures and signs of not-good-enoughness.

The more you recognize that you can't do it all and be it all, and you don't need to either, the more you can turn towards others to help support you and fill the gaps where you lack. We are stronger when we turn towards each other and, despite what we may believe, we are weaker when we try to do everything on our own. Just because you can doesn't mean you should. Just because you get praised for proclaiming, 'I've got this, I'm enough,' doesn't mean that you don't pay the price behind closed doors.

You aren't enough. And rather than hampering your confidence, accepting this truth and beginning to respect your limits can find you more confident, authentic and self-respecting than ever before.

JOURNAL POINTS

1. What is your feeling of not-good-enoughness driven by?
2. What have the costs of striving to be enough been for you?
3. What 'should's are you living by and which ones might you challenge?

———

Not being good enough for the world's standards isn't failure, it's human

7.

People Misunderstand Me

Diving headfirst into the uncomfortable truth

You will feel misunderstood at times when you most need to be seen. You will painstakingly fight your corner, you will desperately try to explain yourself, and people will fail to 'get you'. Feeling misunderstood can make you feel dismissed and ashamed. It's as if life has rewound by decades in a flash and you're just a child crying out to express a need that isn't being met.

You will feel like you're banging your head against a brick wall trying to be understood in circumstances where the cost of being misunderstood might mean losing an opportunity, a relationship or a second chance. You will share your truth with someone with your heart racing and your hands wringing, and they'll say something that indicates that they just didn't understand. You'll feel utterly alone.

Feeling misunderstood can prompt a sense of hopelessness, rage and grief. It can drive friends apart and separate families. It can leave you hauling up the drawbridge of your inner world and swearing never to let anyone step foot inside it again. It's not safe – nobody can be trusted with your secrets, your vulnerability or your hurt. It's just not worth the risk.

As you grow to accept the truth that you will be misunderstood, instead of inspiring you to add some extra bolts to your emotional armour, it actually does the opposite. Accepting that you'll be misunderstood by some people helps you to realize that, in the same way, there will be people who *do* understand, hear, validate, recognize and resonate with how you feel. You'll start to become aware that some people won't 'get you' because they simply can't see where you're coming from, and that's not necessarily to do with you at all, it just means that their life experiences haven't offered them that insight.

Tandia was contemplating ending her long-term relationship and had sought therapy with me to help decide how to go about it and whether it was the correct choice. 'I feel so aware that I want to start a family, but my partner just doesn't want us to have kids. He feels strongly that we'd have a more fulfilled life untethered to the role of parenting and has aspirations to take a transfer overseas and use sabbaticals and annual leave to travel the world.'

Tandia's relationship with her partner was unexpected. He was older than her and she met him through work. They 'never had any of those chats about life plans or hopes' but instead just 'fell hard and fast in a whirlwind relationship', she said. 'I stayed at his house one weekend and basically never left!' He already had two children, whom he had little contact with, so wasn't interested in starting another family and felt he'd 'got the better deal' by not being actively involved in parenting.

'He just doesn't understand me. I grew up in a large family and it's always something I hoped I'd have. Whereas he was an only child and his parents divorced when he was small. He just hasn't experienced, nor does he want to experience, what I had.'

On my recommendation, Tandia and her partner completed a course of couples therapy to chat this through, and both of them felt resolute in their outlooks. Tandia had a difficult decision to make, and after lots of talking and crying (both with her partner and myself), she made the decision to end the relationship. She felt that to give up her potential to become a mother could lead to a feeling of loss and potential resentment towards her partner. 'He didn't get it. And as much as I loved him, there was no way to compromise in this situation and one of us "getting our way" would have harmed our relationship. I needed to be true to myself, even if it meant I had to face the grief of ending something I enjoyed.'

In accepting the uncomfortable truth that you will be misunderstood sometimes, you will be prompted to take more risks in order to find those who do understand you, or in Tandia's case, perhaps some relationships will change as you seek to be understood. What's more, you will recognize that the most important and confidence-boosting thing of all is that *you* understand you.

My story

The feeling of being misunderstood has historically sent me into a tailspin. Remember that moment I picked peanut butter off my jeans at the traffic lights? The feeling I experienced at the woman's disdain was as physical as it was emotional. It felt like panic. There have been a huge number of moments I've felt this way. Suddenly I'd have an overwhelmingly desperate need to put right the misunderstanding, as if my life depended on it.

As I reflected on that moment of panic, I recognized that my response may well have differed from someone else's. Friends of mine wouldn't have responded in such an intense way. They may have rolled their eyes and driven on. As we often say in therapy, when something seems hysterical, it's often rooted in or caused by the historical. My stress survival response was triggered by feeling misunderstood. A real sense of shame would flood me; I'd feel hopeless and helpless. I'd feel like a baby screaming desperately for milk while someone tried to tell me that what I actually needed was a nap.

As I've worked to validate and recognize how the relationship dynamics I experienced with a caregiver as a child led to me feeling unheard and misunderstood, my trauma response has softened. This has changed my life. It means that when I feel misunderstood, I don't automatically rush to my own defence. When I feel like I've tried hard to articulate myself, and someone is committed to not seeing my point of view or acknowledging my side of a story, then I realize that's on them. Understanding that some people don't 'get me' not because they don't care, but because their own life experiences don't allow, just as Tandia found with her partner, has been transformational.

Psychologist Louis Hoffman said of this:

> **self-acceptance too often is intertwined with attempts to rationalize ourselves as being right or justified in our mistakes instead of embracing our humanity as imperfect creatures. Authentic self-acceptance requires that we are honest with ourselves about responsibility. Instead of seeking to justify our mistakes, we embrace them.**

As we begin to separate our self-esteem from how others understand or misunderstand us, then we can start to find a deeper level of self-acceptance.

My work has grown a social media profile and I often receive messages. On the very rare occasion anyone has said anything that makes me feel like my passion-filled work or approach has been misunderstood, I am no longer thrown into a trauma or stress response in the same way. Perhaps it rises up for a moment, but it rarely takes over my day or robs me of sleep as I ruminate all the ways I might get that person to understand me.

Knowing that not everyone will understand me has encouraged me to invest in the relationships and communities I have with those who do. They anchor me. They feed my internal narrative that instead of saying, 'Nobody understands me, I am alone,' now says, 'Not everyone will understand me, and that's okay, because I have people in my life who truly do.'

Why deny?

You know cognitively that some people just won't 'get you'. That would require everyone to have walked the same path and endured the same challenges as you have. It would mean that everyone would have empathy and insight for one another, and we know that this simply isn't

193

true. So why, then, is it so hard to feel okay when you are misunderstood?

- **You've been painfully misunderstood** Like my story, perhaps you also have a story in which you've felt misunderstood or invalidated by a caregiver. The relationship with your caregiver secures your safety and your needs being met in childhood, so any kind of rupture of this relationship can feel painful. An example of this might be that when you feel misunderstood in the present day, you experience feelings of panic or shame because your body and mind are remembering how you felt as a child when a caregiver wasn't able to make you feel valid and understood.

- **Because being rejected impacts survival** Humans are social beings and you need others in order to survive and thrive. This is the reason language was formed, to help people understand one another and communicate. The need to feel understood and like you belong isn't just so that you enjoy the warm and fuzzies, but so that you stay alive in a community. Being misunderstood, therefore, can spark a sense of discomfort for you even if it isn't linked to trauma. This can feed into that drive and need to please others that you explored and reflected on in Chapter 1. Perhaps you recognize that you'd do almost anything to feel understood, liked and accepted by those around you, in order to feel safer. Even if it comes at a high cost to your time, energy and sense of self.

- **You silence yourself to avoid losing something or someone** If you choose to take the risk of explaining your feelings or needs, and someone misunderstands you, you may risk the relationship changing as a result. Perhaps you take the brave step of telling a friend that when they make a certain type of joke about you, it hurts. Perhaps they take offence and, instead of recognizing that you're attempting to protect your friendship, they deflect your words, manipulate your feedback and imply that you should have a better sense of humour. You feel misunderstood and you slowly retreat from spending time with that friend. You decide that, should a similar situation arise, you'll say nothing.

- **You apply significant meaning to being misunderstood** If you lack confidence and self-esteem, it can be harder to risk feeling misunderstood. Perhaps you make shaming statements about yourself in response to someone not 'getting you'. If someone fails to understand you, you conclude that it's your fault for not explaining yourself well enough, or perhaps you shouldn't be feeling how you do. You take responsibility for both what you say and how the other person takes it.

So, seeking to be understood is a survival mechanism of sorts, but the pain you feel when someone misunderstands you is often dictated by the meaning that being misunderstood holds for you. We can't change our human need to be understood by those around us, but there are certainly ways to soften any traumatic response and reduce the need to feel understood by everyone.

The benefits of embracing this uncomfortable truth

If you persist in needing to be understood by those around you, there are many costs to you. However, when you begin to soften towards the uncomfortable truth that you will be misunderstood at times, then there are some really wonderful benefits.

- **Stronger sense of self** As you start to express your needs and opinions in your attempt to be understood, the gap between who you authentically are and the version of you that you portray to others begins to narrow. As you take risks in portraying a more honest version of yourself in an appropriate way within the context you find yourself in, be it in the workplace or with friends, you will strengthen your confidence. Feelings of imposterism will abate and you'll feel more able to work through and with your perceived weaknesses, rather than exhausting yourself by protecting others from them.

- **Release shame** The more you conceal your true self in order to avoid being misunderstood, the more you compound the narrative that there is something wrong and unacceptable about who you really are. Trying to protect yourself from being misunderstood is often an attempt at avoiding shame, when actually it can work to intensify feelings of shame, because you are less likely to experience relationships in which you truly feel accepted and understood.

- **Deeper connection with others** The more you step out in sharing your authentic feelings, opinions and needs, the more likely you are to feel connected to those you share them with. As you take more of an equal space in your relationships, it offers others the opportunity to meet your needs and respect your boundaries in the way you meet and respect theirs. Vulnerability is the antidote to loneliness, because to richly connect with other people you need to feel seen and understood.

- **Treat yourself more kindly** Shame, disconnection and imposter syndrome all contribute to a sense of feeling misunderstood. As you allow yourself to be seen and accepted more by others, this will challenge any lingering, critical internal dialogue and help reinforce a more compassionate relationship with yourself. When you feel accepted by others, it certainly adds weight to the argument that you are acceptable! And the more acceptable you feel to yourself and other people, the more kindly you are likely to treat yourself.

Those are rather huge, life-changing benefits, right? Shame, low self-esteem, loneliness and negative self-talk will soften as you find more acceptance in the truth that you will sometimes be misunderstood. It just goes to show how often we build barriers around the vulnerable parts of who we are in our attempts to protect ourselves. It certainly feels safer, because if you don't speak of your vulnerability and your truth, then nobody can misunderstand or reject it. Sure, those walls keep you safer in some ways, but at the same time they are keeping lots of good stuff out.

As you begin to slowly take these walls down, you open up the possibility for more connection with others, self-kindness and the joy that comes with the freedom to be yourself regardless of whether everyone 'gets you'. Life is riskier outside of those walls, but it's also richer.

Five ways to live with misunderstandings

You want to accept the uncomfortable, freeing truth that you will be misunderstood in life, but those walls you've built to keep you safe from that feeling are hard to tear down. So how do you go about removing the bricks so that you can begin to enjoy the increased confidence and deepened relationships that are beyond them?

1. Accept your vulnerability and step out in vulnerability

What do you think about when you consider the word 'vulnerable'? For me, I used to think about a weak little bird that had fallen out of its nest. It had no strength and relied on others for survival. The more I have come to terms with the fact that my vulnerability, my weaknesses and my needing others is a fact of my humanness and not a failing, the more confident I have grown.

How ironic it seems. The more I accept my weaknesses, the more confident I have become. This is because you have limitations, weaknesses and failings. You always will, regardless of how hard you work on yourself. My client Emma found this acknowledgement hugely liberating. 'For the first thirty-five years of my life I did anything to hide my disability,' she shared. She was born with one arm and felt worried about people treating her differently. 'I didn't want anyone to look at me. I felt ashamed. I'd wear my sleeve right down, and be so conscious if people looked at my prosthetic arm closely.' She was challenged when she needed a new prosthesis made as her old one had worn away where she strapped it on and had become uncomfortable. 'I had to stop wearing it as it was causing pain and I was forced to go about life without it while I waited for my new one.'

However, something brilliant happened. 'I started getting used to people looking at me for a second longer. And as the days went by, it bothered me less. A kid even asked me questions in a queue, and I answered them, thinking that maybe I'd help them understand disability a bit more. My shoulder felt relieved without having the arm strapped on, and I felt much more comfortable physically.' When Emma received her new arm, she was so happy to discover that she didn't even want to use it as she was generally happier without it. 'I know people will look at me sometimes, or be awkward in offering to help me, and I'm becoming okay with that. I've realized how I've done nothing wrong in being born with one arm. I have nothing to hide.' Emma had also begun to follow empowering visible disability accounts on social media and felt bolstered by their confidence in embracing life without hiding their disability. I took great delight in Emma's realization that people only judge what they don't understand.

Like Emma, you don't have to fear people seeing your perceived flaws, weaknesses and failings when you begin to accept that they're a part of you. Often the things we most fear others seeing or knowing are the things we struggle to accept about ourselves.

The more you accept your vulnerability, the less painful it is when people misunderstand it, or can't give you the response you hoped for. To become more accepting of the truth that you'll be misunderstood, you need to give people the opportunity to know you better. This means that, yes, you may well be misunderstood, but you will also have a higher chance of finding those who totally 'get you'.

To put this into action, begin to notice the opportunities that arise to be a little more open and vulnerable. Maybe you could step out in sharing an authentic opinion where usually you'd have nodded along. Perhaps you could ask someone to help you meet a need, such as 'Are you free on Saturday to help me move house?' when previously you'd have struggled along on your own. You'll get more 'no's and maybe even more debates as you express conflicting thoughts and opinions, but you'll also hear more 'yes's and 'Thanks, I hadn't thought of it like that' along the way too. Note down these instances in your journal and see how much easier it becomes in time.

2. Know that some people need to misunderstand you
Some people will misunderstand you because they need to. Over the last couple of years I have challenged my relationship with alcohol. I have let go of my nightly 'treat' of a glass of wine or a gin and tonic, and reduced my consumption drastically. Sometimes I cast my mind back to the years when I believed I needed and deserved my

evening drink. I remember feeling challenged by sober curious posts I saw on social media, or feeling defensive when a friend recommended a book that promoted drinking less alcohol, or shared their experience of abstaining all together.

'Eugh, how judgemental,' I'd think. 'I work hard all day, at work or in parenting, and I deserve my wine. It helps me unwind at the end of the day. I don't get much time to myself; I'll spend it how I damn want.' I wanted to protect my treat and therefore took offence at anything that compromised it or challenged my belief that it was good. To protect my narrative, I needed to misunderstand and reject other people's truth. It doesn't mean they weren't true, or even right or better informed than me, I just wasn't ready to have my truth challenged.

Perhaps you notice that your hackles are up even reading about this! Since I have been open to challenging my narrative, I have become less wedded to my truth and more open to hearing other people's experiences. This isn't me evangelizing about the sober curious life, but an illustration of how I protected myself from a particular narrative. I'm sure that some people felt unseen or misunderstood by me over the years as I held on to my truth. And I'm sure that some people reading this will feel protective over their own narrative, as I share how my own has changed.

My client Ryan was all too familiar with needing to protect his own narrative. 'I stopped seeing my dad when I was nineteen. He had been rubbish throughout my childhood, unkind to Mum and absent with me. Once I left home, I cut him off.' Ryan sought therapy as his dad had been trying to make contact with him at an increasing rate, which had become hard to ignore. He had written Ryan a letter talking about how he'd been having therapy, been clean from drugs for three years and was keen to meet with his son. Ryan had held on to the same narrative about his dad for six years, and it felt challenging to consider that perhaps his dad had changed. 'In my head, Dad was bad. I had felt sad but calmer having chopped him out of my life. It felt simpler, easier. I was done with the drama.'

A few months later, Ryan felt open to meeting his dad for a coffee and came to me to debrief. 'He was different. He was good. He looked well, his face wasn't dark any more. It's going to take me time to trust him, and he said we could take it really slowly, but it felt good to see him.' As Ryan was open to challenging the narrative that had kept him feeling safe for six years, he was giving himself the opportunity to explore a relationship with his dad in a way and at a pace that he felt comfortable with.

I'd encourage you to reflect on any situations in which you've needed to misunderstand or avoid hearing other people's truth in order to protect or preserve your own. In the same way, there will be people in your life who struggle to accept a certain part of your behaviour, your lifestyle or your personality because it challenges something in them that they aren't ready or willing to explore. Sometimes you may be able to have a gentle conversation with someone about this. But often you have to wait until they are ready and open to challenge their own stories and truths. Sometimes you may need to accept the fact that they're protecting themselves from a pain they may never be ready to face.

3. Believe that some people simply don't have the capacity to understand you

It may be that someone misunderstands you simply because they have no idea how it feels to be you, and they aren't able, for whatever reason, to imagine what it feels like to go through a particular challenge you've faced.

My client's house was damaged in a flood. She was having a nightmare dealing with her insurer, and her whole family was displaced to the top floor of her house, surrounded by furniture. She spent the session telling me how difficult it felt as her friend kept complaining about renovation works being done on her house, and how slowly the contractors were working. Jan felt upset and irritated whenever her friend brought this up. She struggled to find patience for their upset, because, well, they should be grateful that they had a dry house at all! She was worried that she had annoyed her friend as she'd cut the conversation short and walked away, boiling with anger. 'She knew what was going on with my home. Why on earth did she feel it was appropriate to drone on about her building works?'

For whatever reason, Jan's friend wasn't able to see beyond her own frustrations to consider how Jan might be feeling. Sometimes we misunderstand each other as humans because our experiences differ so much and life hasn't provided us with the insight, experience or information required to know how to respond to someone in the way they expect and need.

Just because someone doesn't relate to how you feel or they're unable to validate your feelings, it doesn't mean they aren't valid. We often recognize when we compare our situations with others, but do you realize how often you compare your emotions with others? You might think, 'I don't deserve to feel upset, because my friend is having a much harder time than me.' Or, 'I should feel grateful because some people really want what I have.'

You feel how you feel. You are simply having an emotional response to your circumstances. One person may not understand how you feel, but it doesn't mean that someone else won't. Comparing your emotional response to someone else's overlooks the human complexity of why we respond to things the way we do.

We all experience life through our own lenses of experience and understanding. So the best you can do is choose to validate and allow yourself to feel how you feel. Express it, yes, share it and speak it out, yes, but know that you'll be misunderstood along the way. Not necessarily because you don't make sense, but because some people, for whatever reason, can't relate. Keep going until you find those who do.

I encourage you, this week, to find an opportunity to share your experience or feelings and choose to add no meaning or value to how someone responds. It's tricky as we often tend to share things in return for the response we hope will be given. However, in truth, the real value is in your speaking it out. Your response to your circumstances is your response to your circumstances, regardless of whether someone is able to affirm it or not!

4. Seek to understand yourself

As a therapist, light-bulb moments are my favourite thing. Whenever a client proclaims 'I've never thought of it like that' or 'Now that really makes sense', it makes me so happy. It is incredibly helpful to seek understanding of how and why you are the way you are. The more you realize what drives your thoughts, actions and emotions, the more kindness you can offer yourself.

Perhaps through reading this book you've realized that the reason you can be defensive isn't because you're aggressive but because you're protecting yourself from a certain pain or trauma. Maybe you realize that the reason you're irritable around certain people isn't because you're a grumpy character but because you feel misunderstood by them.

We all need to feel understood in order to receive empathy, compassion and a sense of belonging, but if you're finding it hard to extend that to yourself, it can be hard to believe that others might respond to you with kindness and empathy. The more you understand yourself, the more compassion you'll be able to extend to yourself. And the less urgently you need others to understand you. You need to feel understood, so understanding yourself goes part way to meet that need.

My client Alan feared his appraisals each year: 'I would lose sleep for weeks. As the day came, each year I'd vomit before going into work. It was like an annual ritual. My partner would try to encourage me. It literally didn't matter that my appraisals generally went without a hitch, the actual meeting terrified me for some reason.' With his appraisal coming up, Alan wanted to find ways to navigate it differently. We spent time exploring some of the possible reasons he responded to his appraisals in the way he did. We discovered that at school he'd had a science teacher who would 'tear me apart in my report. My parents would shout at me after every parents' evening, and I'd be grounded for some reason or another. I can't even remember what the issue he had with me was, but I don't think the teacher or my parents' reaction was justified.'

As we made connections between his experience of parents' evening and how he braced himself for his appraisal, we began to focus on Alan's 'inner child', who felt terrified at being reprimanded and misunderstood. With this new insight, and sessions focusing on some grounding techniques, Alan's appraisal went much more smoothly than in previous years. He felt anxious and had some disrupted nights, but he didn't vomit beforehand and felt empowered to face the next year's appraisal through this lens.

How, then, do you understand yourself if you feel like you're overreacting and your emotions are spurting out all over the place? Begin to label your feelings. Be inquisitive and not judgemental. Ask what other feeling might be fuelling or mixed in with your reaction?

Once you've acknowledged your feeling, ask yourself what you need. Do you need space, a listening ear, words of comfort or advice? Maybe you need to address an unhelpful habit or implement some new ones that help your well-being. Perhaps you'd benefit from a therapeutic conversation, or making an appointment to speak to a health-care provider for a niggling health issue or trauma. Act upon this need where and when you can. In time, you will find it easier to identify, acknowledge and validate your feelings and, as a result, your thoughts will hopefully feel less tangled and easier to understand.

5. Find people who understand the parts of you that other people don't

You may have people in your life who care about you, but when a certain topic or need arises, they just don't get it. My client Todd had taken up running after doing a Couch to 5k challenge: 'I was never active before. My doctor told me to try to move more after being diagnosed with Type 2 diabetes. Begrudgingly, I downloaded a running app.' Two years later, Todd waxes lyrical about running, crediting it for changing his life. Not only was he off all diabetes medication, he had joined his local running club and signed up to run a half-marathon. Given the many benefits Todd enjoyed from running, he wasn't expecting that his family wouldn't support his new lease of life. 'They laughed at my hobby, calling me obsessed and telling me it was a phase, and they looked forward to it passing so that I'd revert to being the Todd they recognized.'

It hurt Todd that, for some reason, his family found it hard to accept this part of his life that was bringing so much wonderful change. In time, we were able to understand that they struggled to identify with this evolved version of Tod and perhaps were grieving familiarity. We wondered if ridiculing his passion meant they could avoid allowing it to spark positive change in their own lives. The conversations we had meant that, in time, Todd began to accept that perhaps they wouldn't or couldn't understand. And while that was sad for him, he also had people in his community who understood and encouraged him in his passion. It was a shame, but he let go of the need to feel understood by his family in this part of his life, which removed the pressure upon them and alleviated the disappointment he was feeling each time he spoke to them.

Maybe, like Todd, you also feel unsupported by someone in your life who doesn't quite get why something feels so meaningful to you. Perhaps they just don't understand your passion for running, or they find it hard to listen to you enthuse about your job. Maybe they cannot for the life of them imagine why you'd find a certain thing painful, worrying, interesting or angering. They are nice, they are kind, but when it comes to this part of you, you feel alone and misunderstood.

The feeling of 'you just don't get it, you don't get me' softens when you find people who do. When I speak to individuals or engage in communities who have endured traumatic loss as a child, or are juggling parenting and self-employment, I know they understand the nuanced challenges that come with these life experiences.

As a parent, one of my children has specific needs that for a while I didn't see reflected in the families around me. As I spoke of lengthy meltdowns, most parents would smile and say, 'My kid does that too.' But I knew that what we were experiencing was different to what they spoke of and, at times, I felt alone in the challenges that we faced. Despite feeling misunderstood, I decided to continue being honest with people anyway.

Over time, I discovered other parents who were navigating similar challenges, both online and offline. When I'm having a hard time, need advice or am questioning myself, I turn to this handful of people who totally get it. No longer do I feel alone. I might not see my own experience reflected in everyone around me, but I know there are some people who can truly validate and relate to how I feel.

My encouragement to you is that, whatever your situation is, find people who get it. You might have to look a little further, you might have to head online and scour social media to find that pocket of people, but find them all the same – they're out there. Whether it's one friend or a community of thousands, find them.

If you're going through a tough time or grappling with a specific challenge, you might feel 'What's the point in finding people who get it? They can't help me, they can't fix it, they can't take away the feelings or the stress.' If this is your argument, trust me. Perhaps someone might not be able to change your situation, but they can stand beside you as you navigate it. They might not feel your exact emotions, but they can listen to and validate them. They might not be able to be physically there in the tough moments, but you know you're not alone in the feelings that come with them. It's not everything, but it's something. And 'something' when you feel like you've got nothing may well make the world of difference to you.

Conclusion

'People will misunderstand you' – how does it feel to read that uncomfortable truth now after moving through this chapter? If you still feel a squirming discomfort, don't lose heart. It takes time. You may well need to experience more acceptance or to have a few more opportunities to recognize how little someone's misunderstanding of you has anything to do with you at all! Keep searching for your people, keep stepping out in vulnerability, and you'll discover just how liberating accepting this truth can become.

I've earned back time I'd otherwise be spending trying to justify myself. I've removed the pressure from particular people in my life to 'get me' because I've found others who do. I've gained confidence in accepting that I'll be misunderstood and knowing that I can validate my own experience. It will come.

JOURNAL POINTS

1. How do you feel when you are misunderstood?
2. What meaning have you been applying to being misunderstood?

3. Consider who you most feel misunderstood by. Skim over the Five Ways and think about which one you'd like to apply to this relationship or situation.

I can choose to validate my own experiences

8.

Bad Things Will Happen

Diving headfirst into the uncomfortable truth

Bad things have happened to you. Bad things have happened to those you care about. Bad things have happened in this world and are happening right now as you sit reading these words. Someone near you is dying, someone you know is going through heartache, someone is soon to receive a phone call that will make the ground beneath their feet feel like quicksand and change life as they know it. Bad, sad, mad things are going to happen to you at varying intervals for the rest of your life.

You will be on the end of that phone call where time both freezes and speeds up. You will be walking happily down a street and then a car will hit a puddle at just the right angle to drench you. You will lose house keys, jobs, relationships and hopes. And you will do everything in your power to avoid it, but some of the bad things that will happen are stories your busy mind would never even have thought to write.

Your mind will try to pre-empt and protect you from these things happening by playing out the possibilities and potentials at the times you least want it to. When you're trying to get some much-needed sleep you'll imagine a bombshell hitting your life, and as you're contentedly driving down the motorway, a catastrophic crash may play out in your mind's eye.

Perhaps, you feel, if you think of all the things that could go wrong, you'll be prepared and armed when they do. 'Aha,' you'll say, 'I've already lived this through so many times in my head, I know exactly how to ride this out. I've got this figured.' Perhaps you've imagined the feelings that would come along with this sad or bad event so that, if it arises, you'll feel like you've emotionally prepped yourself and it doesn't hurt quite so much as it should because your body and mind have been somehow primed.

Bad things have and will always happen. And if you're wondering how on earth I'm going to help you accept this truth that you spend your time trying to protect yourself from, then read on.

Frieda sought sessions with me to address her emetophobia, an acute fear of vomiting that can be debilitating in day-to-day life and is far more common than people realize. 'Every day I'm scared,' she said. 'Every day I'm jumping when someone coughs in case they're sick, every day I crash into a panic-filled tailspin if someone says they feel unwell or looks remotely off-colour. There are few nights I don't dream about getting a bug and wake up in a sweat.' Frieda lives out her worst fears in her mind, daydreams and nightmares on a daily basis.

In our sessions, Frieda shared how playing through feared scenarios in her head gave her a sense of power and preparedness should they come to fruition. However, over time she began to realize quite how much her phobia was robbing her of experiencing her life to the full as her mind was often elsewhere and her body poised. She also identified how her sleep and general sense of being able to enjoy different situations were impacted by her fear of vomiting.

Over the coming months, along with cultivating a toolbox of techniques to help address the physical effects of her anxiety and to lessen rumination, we spoke in depth about how she has no memories of feeling safe or relaxed for any length of time. Frieda's parents were foster carers and she would often share her home with a child who would have regular physical or loud emotional outbursts. One foster sibling regularly had migraines and would be sick. It made sense to me that Frieda's fragile sense of safety in her own home would somehow become intertwined with the negative association of vomiting. Along with the tools to help her anxiety symptoms, it was so helpful to give voice to 'young Frieda' and affirm the feelings and experiences she'd had as a child that might be presenting themselves in her fear of sickness and her deep desire to protect herself from 'bad things happening'.

Anxiety is often an attempt to pre-empt bad things happening so that we feel some form of control over them. Yet in reality what anxiety tends to do is rob us from being able to enjoy the good things that are happening in our lives and stops us from feeling present in the moment in front of us. Anxiety gives the illusion of protection, whereas actually, in accepting that bad things will happen, we can free up headspace and let go of our attempt to control some of the things that, in truth, we never had control over anyway. In learning to accept the uncomfortable truth that bad things happen, our anxiety is soothed, not fuelled as we might imagine.

Bad things happening can, of course, leave us feeling utterly out of control. Yet contrast this with Viktor Frankl's words in his book *Man's Search for Meaning*, in which he chronicled his experiences in a Nazi concentration camp, saying: 'When we are no longer able to change a situation, we are challenged to save ourselves.' What an acutely powerful encouragement from a man who survived a deeply painful and terrifying experience. Frankl tells us that when we can no longer influence our situation, we must challenge our perspective on it in order to be able to endure it. As you read through this chapter, I hope you will feel more empowered to do the same.

My story

The fear of bad things happening has manifested in so many different ways throughout my life. A common one for me has been staggeringly awful intrusive thoughts that have rocketed into my field of awareness to let me know of the worst-case scenario that could potentially happen in that moment. Think crystal-clear visions of pile-ups happening as I'm driving at 70 mph down the motorway that cause me to white-knuckle grip the wheel and question whether I should divert my route. Think horrifying visions of dropping my baby down the stairs that had my tired mind wondering whether I was fit to be a mother.

For years, until I understood what they were, I was so ashamed of the intrusive thoughts that darted, unprompted, into my mind. Intrusive thoughts are our mind's awareness of risk, possibility, power and responsibility. I might have an intrusive thought about yanking the long ponytail of a fellow commuter on the bus, which raises a cheeky, secret smile at the thought of the chaos that might ensue. However, other intrusive thoughts, far from being amusing, can be disturbing because they deeply conflict with our values and standards of behaviour, which is why they feel jarring and command attention.

It is these harsh or conflicting intrusive thoughts that tend to make us ask 'What do they say about me? Are they things I am capable of?' We wince as a thought flashes into our mind, wondering what on earth people would say if they knew what we were thinking. 'Am I a hazard to myself? Or a hazard to others?'

These days, I know such intrusive thoughts are *just* thoughts, sometimes fuelled by trauma, sometimes inspired by the different potential for risk. Maybe they're an awareness of my responsibility or an acknowledgement of my power to cause chaos or calm. Perhaps they're a recognition of the possibility that lies within every situation for chaos to occur, both within and outside of my control. They're not a reflection of who I am or a statement of what I'm capable of.

So, I still get intrusive thoughts, more so when I'm tired, stressed or hormonal. But I don't turn the 2D thought into a full technicolour theatre any more (well, maybe occasionally). Instead, I notice them and wave them on their way. I'm not in denial that bad things happen – in fact, I feel too fully aware of it sometimes. Is your mind aware of it too? Perhaps you shudder at the busy train station at the image of someone slipping on to the tracks at the worst possible moment. But I can now be quite matter-of-fact about most of the thoughts that hop into my head.

This awareness used to stoke my anxiety like the constant topping-up of coal on an open fire. I remember being shocked that my partner wasn't always considering the worst-case scenario but instead just tended to assume that 'Everything will probably be okay'. I wonder if this comes from my having lived through a 'worst-case scenario' in a way that he hasn't. My voice that reassured me 'Everything will probably be okay' had an echo of 'Yeah, but it once wasn't.'

So, the awareness that bad things could happen used to increase my anxiety, whereas now the acceptance of this very same truth actually eases it! I've tried avoiding bad things, I've spent years imagining what they might be and how they might feel, and it never really made me safer, it just made me tired. As I imagined losing the good things in my life, it tainted my ability to enjoy them while I could. As I tried to control and manipulate situations, and avoided doing things I loved because they involved risk, I didn't feel happier, I felt restricted.

I tried the approach that really helped Frieda address her phobia, and it's serving me very well. If bad things are going to happen, they're going to happen, there's likely to be little I can usefully do to stop them or pre-empt them. I'm going to save my headspace and pre-emptive heartache for when the curve balls actually come. And,

instead, I'm going to use that energy to keep choosing to make the most of the people, the good times and the lovely things that are here within my actual grasp.
While I can.

Why deny?

Why do we work so hard to avoid the uncomfortable truth that bad things do and will happen throughout our lives? And why do we plough so much energy, time and money into the attempt to control our lives in order to prevent bad things happening? And how come, as a result, instead of feeling more at ease, we actually feel more fearful?

- **You know more than ever** Whether you remember life without the internet – phones, search engines that whip up endless answers to any question within milliseconds, a world run by tracked apps – or not, our lives hold increasing unknowns. The more you know, the more questions you'll likely have. The more you know about illnesses you'd otherwise never have heard of, the more potential things you're aware of that could happen to you. You don't want to think about it, but at the same time, you can't stop adding to your repertoire of things to worry about. Perhaps you skim past a news story about political unease. Before you realize it, you're clicking into related news articles and immersing yourself in the contradicting nuances of a sector of politics that moments before you'd had no awareness of. Instead of feeling educated, you feel newly confused, your fear and anxiety rising at what this may mean for your life and income.

- **Anxiety feels familiar and productive** Anxiety and worry, as much as you find it frustrating, can become a coping mechanism. It can become the background buzz to your life, the static you're so used to that you forget to question whether it needs to be there. Sometimes rumination over bad things happening fills the space in your mind so that you can avoid feeling sadness, for example. Anxiety can feel productive and protective in a world of unknowns.

- **You've experienced trauma and self-protection** If you have endured a traumatic life experience, then you may well do everything you can in order to protect yourself from going through something bad again. Whether you find yourself withdrawing from relationships a little bit or your mind totally fixating on avoiding a certain risk, unaddressed trauma makes bad things feel like a collective of experiences that you could never endure again.

- **Safety-seeking behaviour feels . . . safe** You only do things that feel safe. Perhaps you are worried about traffic accidents so you don't drive. Maybe you feel worried about people judging you, so you avoid group events. Safety-seeking behaviour means you are less likely to face your fears, because it feels safe, despite how small and limited it makes your world.

- **You don't complete the circle of emotion** If you fear certain emotions such as grief or anger, you may do everything you can to protect yourself from feeling them. Distracting, numbing, denying, invalidating – there are so many ways you can try to avoid your feelings. But, as a result, you don't move through the grief or the anger and come out the other side. You don't have enough experience of the truth that you can allow yourself to feel grief and notice how it lessens in time to make way for acceptance. Or that the anger will pass to make way for calm. The avoidance of certain emotions fuels the narrative that bad things cause scary feelings that may never ease off.

Safety feels like a good thing to pursue, doesn't it? Surely it's not wise to let your guard drop and live a risky life with little regard for rules and regulations? Of course, it's good to be safe. When self-protection is driven by common sense, that's . . . sensible. Wear the seat belt, hold the guard rail, don't eat stuff that smells bad. But the self-protection I'm alluding to here is the anxiety-driven self-protection – the times you do or avoid certain things because something bad might happen, when actually the experience could bring so much joy and enrichment.

I didn't drive for ten years due to driving anxiety and preoccupation with crashes. Millions of people drive each day, regardless of the risk it holds. It's safer not to drive, granted, but my reticence was fuelled by an anxiety that limited my life. So, as you continue through this chapter, hold in mind the self-protective behaviours and decisions you make that limit your life in some way, those driven by fear and anxiety regardless of how much risk is actually involved.

The benefits of embracing this uncomfortable truth

Holding up a battle shield to defend yourself when arrows are being flung at you is protective. Holding up that battle shield permanently and preventatively, just in case someone comes to fight you one day, is exhausting. But as you begin to embrace the uncomfortable truth that bad things will happen, you can opt to do other things with that energy. You realize there are so many beautiful things to see beyond that shield. The avoidance of the uncomfortable truth that bad things will happen often involves a great urge to protect ourselves, yet opening up to the truth helps you ease into more acceptance of the fact that there are some things you simply cannot control. Here are some benefits you'll experience as you do so.

- **Reduces anxiety** Anxiety is an inbuilt, life-saving, nervous system response. When you become aware of danger, your body responds with a rush of hormones that rev your body up to fight or flee. This is all well and good when you're faced with physical threat, but when you fear bad things happening all the time, it's likely that your body and mind are responding with spiralling, frantic thoughts and a racing heart that make it hard to rest and feel present. As you spend less time focusing on the possibilities of bad things happening, you'll enjoy a calmer nervous system and mind.

- **Fewer intrusive thoughts** The more you fear bad things happening, the more hypervigilant and on guard you will be. You may experience intrusive thoughts, those anxiety, fear-based images that pop into your mind and alert you to a worst-case scenario. These thoughts can be fuelled by unaddressed trauma, and they can be unpleasant. As you choose not to apply so much time, meaning and focus to those thoughts, you are more likely to prevent the anxiety spiral they cause.

- **Unlimited enjoyment of the good things** It is hard to enjoy things when your mind is focusing on what could go wrong in that moment. As you choose to stop ruminating over all the negative possibilities, your mind and body are more present, available and able to enjoy the moment and all the beauty that lies within it.

- **Seize opportunities and experiences** As you stop bracing yourself for something bad to happen, you are more likely to feel able to engage in the experiences that lie in front of you. Fear of something going wrong will become less of a deciding factor in the choices you make, leaving you open to new experiences in life that may well involve a healthy, empowering dose of risk!

- **You stop trying to control the things you cannot control** Trying to control the outcome of different scenarios keeps you living small and tired. As you focus on the things within the realm of your control rather than those outside of it, you tap into the rather uncomfortable but potentially very freeing sense of 'going with the flow' where you can. You're more likely to throw yourself into life, which is risky in its essence regardless of what you do or don't do, and can reap the benefits of engaging in it fully rather than tirelessly tiptoeing around possibilities.

In order to live a full and thriving life, you must live a risky one. In order to have more fun and life experience, I needed to get behind the wheel of my car and drive beyond my postcode. In order to have the life-enriching experience of loving and being loved, I needed to risk heartbreak. A good life is inevitably a risky one because, if we are honest, it is safe but a little boring within our comfort zones.

So then, how do you move from fearing that bad things will happen to accepting that bad things will happen and live a fuller life as a result?

Five ways to live with the truth that bad things will happen

Here are my five tips to help you move from that place of fear to acceptance.

1. Know you've survived so far

You, right now, have survived every bad thing that has ever happened to you. Every challenge you've faced that made you think 'I can't do this', you did. You moved through it and came out the other side. Perhaps you're reading this from the midst of a messy or painful time, questioning whether you'll ever make it through. Look at the proof by looking backwards, consider the different curve balls you've endured, heartache that has healed, the pain you've lived through or learned to live with.

You might be bruised and battleworn, but you're here. My client Felicia began therapy to deal with the loss of her long-term partner. She, like everyone I work with in the depths of grief, questioned whether she'd ever feel happy again: 'Will I ever laugh properly? Like when my side hurts from my laughter and nothing else in the world matters? Will I live a day without lugging around this horrible, dark weight of sadness?' And the answer is always

'Yes'. I encouraged Felicia in the same way I encourage others, and in the same way I've had to encourage myself too. There is hope: we see it in the faces of those we've watched walk through the pain of loss, we've heard it in the stories of those who have rediscovered happiness that grows like roots around a stone. We've got our own stories that we can reflect on to affirm this truth too.

I remember dark days of depression. One day I walked in the rain, feeling like the sky was crying along with me. I spoke to my mother on the phone. 'There will be light at the end of the tunnel,' she said. 'But when?' I pleaded. I needed to know exactly when the light would pour in. She couldn't say. But she was right, it did. I moved through the tunnel of depression, plodding forward in the risks I took in sharing my feelings. I lifted one heavy, tired foot in front of the other each time I let someone's kindness challenge my inner bully. Just as my client Felicia experienced, it was as if the tunnel's concrete started cracking. Little streams of light made their way through, casting a glow on the dust. Slowly, the tiny ribbons of light gave way to beams as the sunshine broke through.

I have been changed by each period of darkness, each stressful time, each curve ball that hit, each moment I've

questioned whether I've got it in me to make it through.
And so will you.

If you need some actionable encouragement right now,
remember that sometimes you have to look back in
order to motivate yourself to keep moving forward.
Consider your own experiences of pushing through, of
seeing the sun stream into dark seasons again, of
laughing after it feels like sadness or darkness has
prevailed for too long. Keep feeling, keep validating,
keep leaning on others. Use your past survivals, big
and small, as proof that you can and you will make it
out the other side. Seek the stories of others who have
endured hard times and found a way to live and
laugh again.

2. Address anxiety-fuelling trauma

So, you've endured many different challenges and stresses
through life and, as I say, you've survived. But to what
degree? You might be physically alive, but perhaps your
heart feels perpetually broken; perhaps as much as you
try, you cannot drop the shield despite the fact that your
muscles are burning and your hands are blistered. You
are alive, but in some ways you're not actually living,
you're stuck.

A client of mine spent time addressing his agoraphobia (fear of leaving a safe environment, which, for Luke, meant his home). He was so proud to have reached a place where he'd confidently, without panic or anxiety, head out to work and run necessary errands. He loved his newfound freedom, yet felt that something was still missing: 'I am so glad to be where I am now, but I never imagined I'd feel so lonely. I thought everything would be better when I found ways to manage my panic attacks and get to work again.' Together we discovered that while Luke was enjoying the progress he'd made, over the years his social life had dwindled to nothing as friends stopped visiting him. He could leave his home, but the feelings of isolation were still there. A few weeks later, Luke reignited his old hobby of cycling, dusted off his bike and joined a local club. In time, not only had he regained his freedom, he had new friendships which increased his sense of well-being and connection.

When you've been through a hard time or trauma, you may have recovered enough to be here to tell the tale, but your quality and enjoyment of life haven't recovered fully. This tells us that either you're still walking through it and processing what you've been through and endured, or you've got stuck in that tunnel and you aren't able to move forward any more. You can see there's a route, and everyone tells you to keep on keeping on and 'you're doing great', but you can't muster the energy or coordination to keep walking. Maybe you just don't know how.

Pause right here. Do you feel like you're stuck in that tunnel? If so, what do you need? You need people to support you as you trudge through to the exit. To hold the torches, to let you lean on them so they can relieve you of some of the weight. That's not failure, it's just that sometimes the things we go through are too big, too complicated or too messy for one person to bear. Find support, online or offline, make an appointment or a phone call (see the Helpful Contacts section at the back of the book), or open up to a friend. Perhaps you acknowledge that you've emerged safely through a dark time, but things don't feel quite right. Consider what is missing for you. Is it connection? Perhaps you'd benefit from acknowledgement of your challenging time or ideas for how to venture forward. How might you take a step onwards to meet a need or two and find your confidence in this new season?

Trauma disrupts your sense of safety and can make it hard to move out of a state of hypervigilance. You can find yourself living as if on high alert, poised and ready for something else to happen. With the right support, the experiences you went through can move from lurching about in your awareness as an almost constant reminder that life isn't safe, to being stored in a different part of your brain where it has less power over your day-to-day. With the right support, in time, you can feel safe again.

3. Arm yourself with tools to stop anxiety spiralling

Imagine standing at the roadside and watching the cars pass by. You cannot control or predict which colour car or lorry will come into your line of vision next, but you can choose not to flag one down and climb inside. In the same way, you can observe any thoughts that pop into your head, but in time you can learn to stop them from taking hold and spiralling to the extent that your fight-or-flight stress response kicks off. I'm going to give you some tools in a moment to help you halt the spiralling thoughts.

Anxiety is that life-saving, inbuilt mechanism there to keep you safe. Animals at a watering hole, on hearing a distant lion roar, will suddenly be fuelled with adrenaline. They pause from contentedly drinking the water. Their ears prick up to assess the roar and risk, their muscles are poised and ready to run or fight for their lives. The volume of the roar lessens, the risk is next to none. They are safe. Their sympathetic nervous system recedes along with the adrenaline and vigilance, and they resume drinking the thirst-quenching water.

In an ideal world, this is how your anxiety would function. It would rise at risk and then recede as the risk passes. The challenge comes when your anxiety is triggered often, or by thoughts of bad things happening that don't come to fruition. Your body simply cannot take the risk of assuming that the worst-case scenario your mind is considering is not happening. If a fire alarm goes off when you're in a supermarket, you can't just assume it's a false one, everyone has to go through the motions and file outside until given the all-clear.

Now imagine how exhausting it would be if you worked in that supermarket and the alarm went off all the time! This is how anxiety works when our body constantly responds to our spiralling thoughts. Anxiety is one of my favourite things to work with in the therapy room. This is because it's so possible, with the right tools, for clients to find a new sense of confidence and safety in their circumstances. One of my clients described in such a brilliant way how it felt to address their feelings of anxiety: 'When I came for therapy it felt like I was on a plane constantly braced for impact. Not literally, but this is how living day-to-day felt for me. I was tense and ready to protect myself. After a few sessions, it was like my body and mind unfurled from that brace position and I was able to enjoy snacks and books like my other fellow flyers!'

So, yes, I love working with anxiety because there is a boatload of hope. I have so much to say about anxiety that I could write an entire book on the topic (in fact, I wrote one about postnatal anxiety called *Mind Over Mother*). Here are some tools to try in order to help yourself when you feel anxious:

- Ask yourself what you're feeling and needing in the moments you feel 'okay'. Tending to your needs and feelings can help slow or prevent the build-up into anxiety.
- When you notice that you're feeling anxious, ask yourself what you're fearing. What can you do to challenge the anxious thought or meet the need beyond it?
- To halt rumination, count back from 100 in threes and use a simple breathing technique to calm your body. Try a deep inhale for 4 and an extended, full exhale for 7.

- When you feel your fight-or-flight response kick in, do something physically active such as star jumps or jogging on the spot. This utilizes the flood of adrenaline!
- Find a mantra. I like 'I will cross that bridge if I get to it'. It's a reminder that not only do half the things I fear never come to fruition, but I have crossed many bridges of challenge in the past and made it to the other side.

4. Fatigue the fear and let go of control

I remember the day I decided to change tack in the way I approached my fear of bad things happening. Instead of trying to reassure myself that 'it will be fine', when a huge part of me didn't believe that little sentence, I tried thinking about it in a different way. 'Bad things will happen,' I repeated to myself, like a wonky, dysfunctional affirmation. I repeated it in my mind in moments when I felt peaceful and content. I said it out loud as I walked around my home on work days.

It sounds doom and gloom but, actually, I began to fatigue the fear. I began to accept it as a fact beyond my control, rather than an anxiety-fuelled sentence that had me grappling for that same control. The phrase 'Bad things will happen' became less barbed as I continued to repeat it.

The other thing that really helped was to make conscious choices to soften my focus on the outcome of everything, to try to find some more ease in the unknown.

One of my favourite tips to help put this into action is this: if you have a stressful morning, try not to assume that you're going to have a bad day. Let the day reveal itself along the way and perhaps you'll see some of the good within it, rather than looking for the stress that affirms your prediction.

My client Gloria found this particularly helpful and shared this in our session: 'Most days I'd wake up in a bad mood, and then find myself stomping through my day. I'd say, "Great, another bad day." After we spoke, I stopped saying that to myself, and my family, and I tried to just see what happened as the day went on. I realized that by saying it was a "bad day" I was more likely to have a bad day. I tried not to drag how I felt one hour into the next hour, and it was brilliant! My days were more "mixed" than "bad" or "good".' I loved witnessing Gloria enjoy seeing what happened when she chose not to make powerful blanket statements about her whole day.

Challenge yourself to sit with the little unknowns in order to train you up for the bigger unknowns of life. You don't really know what will happen tomorrow; you can make a good guess and you can plan each minute with precision, but ultimately what will happen will happen. If dwelling on this uncertainty feels uncomfortable and inspires anxiety, then try leaving some small questions unanswered. Next time you reach for the phone to do a web search for the weather or the answer to a trivia question, try letting it be. Next time you wonder how an old friend from college you've not spoken to in ten years is doing, let it be. Next time you feel an urge to check a friend isn't mad with you for that boundary you just asserted, let it be.

This is a gentle way to become more acquainted with the unknown. In a world that encourages us to seek mastery over every area of our life and leave no question unanswered, this takes some strength. Especially if your phone is sitting nearby winking at you! Embrace the ancient, mind-expanding practice of 'wondering': *I wonder what the weather will be like. I wonder what that old friend is up to. I wonder if this afternoon will feel more balanced than this morning.* If anxiety is about seeking control, 'wondering' is about holding the reins more loosely. Caring about the outcome and worrying about the outcome are two different things, and neither have any bearing on the outcome itself!

5. Choose to let the storm pass

Storms pass on their own regardless of how we wish them along. No man-made machine would hurry the storm past faster or hold it back. It is far beyond our realm of control. We can only look at the sky and watch it roll in.

Tough times are those storms in your life. You can batten down the hatches, you can ensure you've got food to last the storm, but you can't control where the storm goes or when it ends. However, you sure can spend a lot of energy, time and stress trying to guess and obsess. A brittle tree is more vulnerable to the storm whereas one that bends and flexes is more likely to weather it.

One particularly challenging day, two of my kids were upset over dropped ice creams in the high street. One lay flailing on the floor. I couldn't carry both her and my shopping. Once, I might have begged, bribed and blushed as people walked by: 'Please, come on, I'll get you another, we need to get to the car, please stop, everyone's looking at us.' I've worked out that these tactics don't really usher the storm along, but the trying and the pleading just add pressure and stress. So, on that day, I sat on the pavement in the dust and waited for the storm to pass. It did. As it always does.

Where are you trying so hard to usher along a tough time, when actually your energy would be better preserved by simply doing what you can do and then buckling up for the ride? Sam was waiting for a biopsy result. He came to one session and shared how he'd 'exhausted the internet' reading about every possible outcome. He'd been on the phone to the hospital multiple times a day hoping for the results. We explored some ideas that would help him preserve some of this energy and feel more supported as he navigated the unknown. He decided to limit his calls to one per day and pledged to try not to research further, which had only fuelled his anxiety. He also decided he'd meet a friend the following day to seek support in the waiting.

It's hard living in the unknown, but we live in it all the time. Often, we just believe we have control, but in truth we have far less control than we like to think. As you choose to loosen your grip, calm your anxiety and bring balance with presence, you're opting for acceptance over fear.

Conclusion

Don't let your life be a waiting room for bad things happening. It's like opting to live in a tiny underground war bunker before you've even heard the sirens sound.

Bad things will happen, but not all the time. And along the way some rather wonderful things will happen too. Use gratitude to help you recognize the incredible things that exist in the beautiful, boring day-to-day. Boring itself is a gift for it is devoid of drama! Even in the blackest rubble, you'll find the rubies if you look hard enough.

They say that life is like a roller coaster, but I disagree. There is always something good running alongside something tough, meandering and weaving through your life if you're open to seeing it. People have walked through your deepest fears and are thriving. People have faced challenges they didn't even know were possible and they've navigated them. And, if required, you will too. You don't know what's around the corner, but don't let the fear of the potential rob you from living your today. Lean into the unknown, befriend it.

It's amazing how empowered you can become as you get acquainted with your powerlessness.

JOURNAL POINTS

1. How has your anxiety been both serving and costing you?
2. What fears fuel your anxiety? Which tools might you try?
3. In what area of your life might you encourage yourself to ease the reins of control a bit?

———

Good things happen too

9.

I Will Lose People I Love

Diving headfirst into the uncomfortable truth

Do you know what? When I wrote this book, I had this big, uncomfortable truth down as Chapter 2. On reflection, I moved it all the way to the end of the book because I realized it's such a hard hitter and I wanted you to feel like you could trust that I would approach it gently and give you a boatload of hope along the way. As we now dive into the uncomfortable truth that you will lose some of those you love – the truth that fuels anxiety and nightmares – I hope you know you're in good hands.

If you haven't already walked through the fire of grief, you will. If you haven't already lost someone that you love, someone who you don't believe you could live without, you will. Tragedy will touch you somehow, whether something happens to someone close to you or you live on the periphery of someone else's pain.

This uncomfortable truth fuels our nightmares and has us bracing ourselves when loved ones board flights or await test results. Loving others makes us feel vulnerable and young. We cannot help but allow our hearts to invest in the life and hearts of others. People are meaningful to us, even though we sometimes attempt to put up our guards in order to protect ourselves from the pain of loss.

I'm fully aware that this uncomfortable truth pervades many sleepless nights, and is the cause of heartache and anxiety, much as it is my own. But throughout this chapter I am going to help you see it differently. Instead of fear, this truth will prompt intentionality, empowering you to make the most of the good relationships in your life. I will reframe the anxiety around loss to inspire a warm sense of gratitude and contentment that both softens the anxiety and sits beside it.

I think this was so beautifully encapsulated by my client Linda's words. Linda had begun therapy as a way to deal with the loss of her mother. 'I had seen my own grandmother lose herself through grief when she lost her mother and I didn't want to do that too.' Linda's mother had explained that her grandmother withdrew from her relationships as a response to her grief, hoping to protect herself from any pain of potential loss.

'Losing Mum was the most painful thing that has ever happened to me,' Linda told me. 'But, throughout my life, she helped me realize that there was always good to be found in hard times. As a child she'd encourage me to look for the leaf buds on trees that seemed dead, or point out a nice cloud formation in a dark sky.' This practice had been such a legacy for Linda as she walked the path of grief. 'So many see life like a roller coaster of highs and lows, but I don't,' Linda shared. 'I see it like a winding train track, where the good and the tough sit side by side. Some of my days have been horribly dark and painful, but there have always been beautiful things within them. Sometimes I have to open my eyes wider, or look harder, but I always see them.'

Death is the conclusion of all life, just as grief is the price we pay for experiencing the richness of love. And if we, like

Linda, can choose to be open to the beauty amidst the sadness and challenges of life, both in the hard times and the stressful moments, it might be painful, but it's not all painful. It might be hard, but it's not all hard. And grief might be the price we pay for love, but we can stop the fear of loss from robbing us of the opportunity to revel in that love where we can.

My story

One night, my partner was due home late after an event at work. I lay awake wondering why he hadn't arrived when he said he would. His phone wasn't ringing through and, from what I could see on my app, the train he was due to get had run on time. My wondering slid into anxiety. My heart picked up pace as I began to imagine that his Tube train had crashed or been blown up. I couldn't lie still as I questioned how I'd break the news to our three children. How would I pay the mortgage? Would I need to move in with my parents? Did I know all the logins to cancel our utilities? My body responded to my spiralling thoughts as if the tragedy were living truth, rather than a desperate story written by my imagination. My heart physically ached at the thought of grief, my body tense with despair.

Shortly after, he crept into the room, questioning why I was starkly awake. He'd missed his train and his phone had run out of charge. As he slipped into sleep, the adrenaline still coursing through my veins pushed my own rest out of reach.

The fear of losing someone I love is the main theme of my anxieties. I have two types of hugs that I give those I love: the kind that speaks of 'I'm so grateful to have you in my life' and the white-knuckle hugs that say 'I am so afraid to lose you'.

In my journey of facing the uncomfortable truth of inevitable loss, I have found that my anxiety has softened. I have lost less sleep through fear and enjoyed more of the 'I'm grateful for you' hugs. Moving towards a place of acceptance of the truth that I have spent a lifetime running from prompts me to be more intentional and present in my relationships. Staying more conscious of the uncomfortable truth of loss means that I'm more likely to opt for a moment on the sofa with my loved ones over an extra few seconds spent dashing around doing jobs about the house. It means I'm more likely to linger over a wonderful view, instead of my eyes continually darting to my watch to ensure I'm bang on time. A healthy awareness of loss, rather than avoidance, invites me to make choices that ensure I live a little more aware of what's going on around me. It invites me to slow my pace and my breath, and to be a bit more of a human 'being' rather than my tendency to spend every waking moment as a human 'doing'. We need to be both, of course, but many of us would benefit from a little more 'being'. Let's move you towards that place too.

Why deny?

On the face of it, it seems quite obvious as to why we'd choose to avoid the uncomfortable truth that we will lose people we love. We don't want to think about it because it's painful. It sends waves of anticipatory grief through our core. It's too hard to even go there. Yet we do. We go there in our anxieties, right? We don't want to face it, yet the fear sits below the surface of love, waiting to be disturbed or nudged by a story we hear about someone else's loss, or an announcement that someone is missing a work day due to a funeral. Hearing about loss prompts thoughts about loss. Loving others prompts awareness of loss.

We don't want to think about it, but we do. So, if we are going to think about it regardless of whether we wish to or not, why not come to peace with it a little more? In finding a different way to approach this uncomfortable truth, we can come to a fresh acceptance of the risk and inevitability of loss in our lives. And as we begin to accept it, we find a way to live with it.

Living with an accepting awareness of the fact that we will lose those we love is far better than using a huge amount of energy fighting the fear that crops up in our nightmares and follows hot on the heels of our feelings of love and gratitude. In *A Matter of Death and Life*, the psychiatrist Irvin Yalom shares how he navigated the cancer diagnosis and subsequent death of his wife, Marilyn (along with her own reflections). He writes 'mourning is the price we pay for having the courage to love others'. To wish for a life without mourning and sadness is ultimately to yearn for a life devoid of love.

So, yes, we do what we can to stop thinking about loss because it's painful. Yet to find acceptance may well enable us to engage more freely with the opportunities to experience love in our lives. Before we explore how to do this, let's look at some of the reasons you might avoid accepting the truth that you'll lose those you love.

- **You've not seen someone journey through healthy grief** Perhaps you haven't witnessed someone move through the process of grief in a way that feels both honouring of their experience of loss and progressive towards a place of acceptance, building in time to a fulfilling life in full awareness of the loss, rather than avoidance of it. Or maybe you've observed someone respond to their grief through numbing, addiction or abuse. Both of these experiences could fuel the belief that losing someone you love is too great a pain to live with, that life changes beyond all recognition and there is little chance of rebuilding it.

- **You've learned to be anxious about loss** When we are young, we look to our caregivers to tell us about the world. Perhaps your caregiver struggled with acute anxiety around the death of loved ones. Maybe adults in your life made decisions about your safety that felt restrictive, but were driven by fear of losing you. For example, my client Laila's mother would message her incessantly whenever she took a long journey. After losing her own sister to a road traffic accident, Laila's mother needed constant reassurance that Laila was safe. 'As an adult in my forties, this can feel a bit overbearing,' Laila told me. 'I understand her anxiety, but at the same time, I do feel like she'd benefit from some therapy as her constant focus on losing me has definitely fed into my anxiety around driving because at times I felt it'd be better for her and safer for me if I never drove at all.' Perhaps, like Laila and her mother, you may have felt that your fear-fuelled attempts to control what happens around you is what keeps you or a loved one safe.

- **Death is a taboo in many cultures** In Western culture, talking about death can feel taboo. Unlike the practice in other cultures, bodies are generally whisked away and hidden from those grieving. The very avoidance of a topic reinforces the taboo. And where there is taboo, there is fear, mystery and confusion. This makes it difficult to talk about loss and tough to know how to approach and support those grieving; risking that loss looks like a lonely, shameful journey.

- **We are taught to numb and avoid pain** As children, many of us were encouraged to divert our emotion or attention away from unpleasant things.

'Don't cry, you're okay,' we may have been told as we shed tears as a toddler. Or 'Be grateful, most teenagers don't have what you have,' we may have been told as we expressed discomfort as a teen. This continues into adulthood. A twinge? Take a pill. A tough day? Grab a drink. Bored? Drown out the silence with music. Sad? Embark on a TV binge. There are unending ways to numb and avoid pain in our society, so it's no wonder we seek to avoid thinking about loss. But, in reality, we think about it anyway. Numbing and avoidance mean we don't process or make space for our fears and feelings, which are the best ways to address them.

- **You've endured traumatic loss** If you have endured loss that has been traumatic in any way, then unaddressed trauma fuels ongoing anxiety. Trauma lurches into your line of vision and the pain simmers just beneath the surface of every situation you face. It's hard to reassure yourself that it could possibly be survivable to lose someone again when loss has so deeply pervaded so many areas of your life and you feel traumatized.

- **Death challenges important structures in your life** You might especially fear someone's death if your identity is enmeshed with theirs. Perhaps they are the one person in your support network or their advice and encouragement is the only source you have to turn to. Perhaps they feel like the linchpin to everything that feels safe and familiar in your life, so if you lose them, you lose yourself somehow.

As tough a topic as this is to dive into, I wonder if you have gained some new clarity as to why this uncomfortable truth is so hard to accept. Understanding why it's tough for you helps you know where you might need extra support, therapeutic insight or kind words in order to take some of the sting out of the fear. When we understand the truth of why we fear loss so much, we can open our mind to the fact that perhaps we could grow in our acceptance of the inevitable.

The benefits of embracing this uncomfortable truth

Before I share with you five ways in which to grow in acceptance of the inevitability of loss, let's take a closer look at some of the freeing benefits of choosing to accept the inevitable truth that you will lose someone you love.

- **Deeper connection with others** I remember wishing that I never loved anyone as it would prevent the pain of loss. As soon as you seek to keep yourself safe by holding back from relationships, you are risking missing out on much-needed connection with others. Humans are hardwired for connection, and letting yourself love others and be loved requires vulnerability and openness. As you grow in acceptance of loss, it paves the way for more deep, meaningful and safe relationships.

- **Reduced anxiety** Death is at the core of many anxieties and phobias. You may fear losing others, so you seek to control your life and avoid risk. Anxiety gives you the illusion of control, yet in reality you can feel out of control as thoughts spiral. As you soften towards the inevitability of losing others, this means that anxiety won't taint as many of your interactions and thoughts, leaving you with valuable headspace and the opportunity to lean into the moment.

- **Preserve energy from trying to control the uncontrollable** When anxious about loss, you often seek to keep people safe. This can lead you to making decisions that can feel restrictive, such as 'Oh, don't drive that far, get the train' or 'No, it's dangerous to go to that country, stay closer to home'. As you accept that you cannot control everything, you will feel less of an urge to invest energy and time and potentially impact relationships in seeking to control different variables and outcomes.

- **Less guilt in relationships** The fear of loss might fuel a sense of guilt that you aren't making the most of those you love. You may apply pressure on yourself that you should always be 'doing more'. A little guilt can prompt you to take action and to connect with those you care about, but as you let go of excess guilt and pressure, you are more freed up to enjoy your interactions with others.

- **Connect in the present moment** Just as in those white-knuckle, anxiety-filled hugs I mentioned, when you veer into fear of loss rather than acceptance that it's a part of life, your mind runs into a future that has not yet happened. Anxiety takes you out of the moment and into a place of fear. Seeking to find more peace with the uncomfortable truth of loss invites you to breathe in and be more present in the moments that are happening right in front of you.

I'm sure that you'll be able to add further benefits to my list, and if more have come to mind, make a note of them in the margin or your journal. There is a cost to love; there is a price to pay for the joy that relationships bring. And choosing to find slow acceptance of the reality of life's risk means that you won't hold back from loving and living more wholeheartedly when given the opportunity.

Five ways to live with the truth that you will lose those who you love

1. Know that people have survived grief

Of course you know that grief is survivable, you see people living and grieving. Perhaps it is possible to die of a broken heart, as some elderly people are known to slip away shortly after the loss of their lifelong partner. But what I mean here is surviving in the sense of truly living. You may have known someone who, while still alive, actually seemed to die along with their loved one. Unprocessed grief and traumatic loss, as we've touched on, can leave people stuck, feeling as if the loss happened yesterday.

But when grief is allowed and accepted, when there is no dam built against the feelings that come in waves, whatever they may be, then people certainly can and do thrive after loss. People have thrived after walking through the fire of your nightmares. People have survived grief. People have thrived after loss, trauma and tragedy.

One day, I stumbled across the story of a woman who had recently lost her partner. She was in the thick of grief. I threw myself into her story, as we often do, and felt intensely fearful that I would also be widowed. Later that day, I found myself on social media and accidently found a woman who had started a business in supporting widows through loss, empowering them to build full and happy lives. She was smiling, telling her own story of how, with the right support, she was well. I look at my mother too, someone who has lived through my deepest fear of losing a child. She is changed, and a part of her will always be deeply aware of who is missing in her life, but she is thriving.

My encouragement to you is to seek out a couple of stories of those who have continued to build a full life around their loss to give you a sense of hope that, with the right support and tools, you could do the same. This is a sturdy reminder that there is a healthy future beyond loss and heartbreak. It helps bring a balanced understanding of

how loss feels and makes the truth that you'll lose
someone a little less fear-filled.

2. Be intentional about your relationships and where you invest your energy

Take a moment to write down a list of those most
important to you, the ones you wish you spent more time
with. These may be the people you feel sadness and guilt
about when you don't see them for a length of time.

You only have limited resources of time and social
energy. I often find myself filling my weekends and then
feel a pang as I realize we overlooked the opportunity to
see our parents. If you feel these little pangs and aches,
let them guide you towards making time for those who
mean the most to you. Life will flood into the blank
spaces in your diary and sometimes we need to ring-
fence time with those we wished we saw a little
more often.

My client Irsa lost her mother suddenly in her twenties.
She felt plagued by the thought that she might lose her
father, who lived abroad, before she got to see him again.
As a result, she kept travelling the lengthy journey to see
him multiple times a year, which was beginning to have an

impact on her work and family life. 'I can't face the thought that he might die like my mother, and I'll just get a call and be far away,' she told me. As we worked together to help her process the trauma of losing her mother so suddenly, ten years before, Irsa felt able to reframe how she saw her visits to her father.

Instead of booking flights frantically after having a bad dream or an anxious day, in time she learned to manage her anxiety and mother herself through moments of grief. Her visits became less frequent, but when she did spend time visiting her father it felt different: 'It was less adrenaline-filled. As I hadn't had to scramble for sudden leave from work, it meant it was less guilt-filled too. The other thing that felt different was that I could have better boundaries with work as I was taking proper annual leave instead of suddenly disappearing and feeling like I had to show I was still working.' For Irsa, spending more intentional and planned time with her father meant that the quality felt much more enjoyable for both of them. Spending time with someone out of fear of losing them has a different quality to when we find tools to quell our anxiety and manage to be just a little more present (turn to the end of Chapter 8 to find some of my favourite tools for lessening anxiety).

At one point I was only seeing my own father about once every four months. I live a full and fast life with three kids, and weekends are dominated by their clubs and events. Though my mother would come to look after the kids at times, he would often stay home. I had a moment of stark awareness that if he lived to seventy-five, for example, then perhaps I would only see him around another twenty times in his life. Wow.

In facing and pondering the truth that one day, unless I die first, I will lose him, I felt prompted to be more intentional about seeing my parents together.

As you allow your mind to acknowledge the truth that you will lose people you love, you can move towards those people a little more. Perhaps your diary is full of things and people that, in truth, don't matter as much to you. You can choose to be more selective with where you place those limited resources of time and social energy in order to make a bit more space for those few precious people.

3. Arm yourself with tools for anxiety

When your imagination is weaving a tale of tragedy and loss, your body responds. You feel your heart race and your adrenaline levels soar. This is because your nervous system simply has to believe that what you are thinking is happening. What you experience is your sympathetic nervous system lurching into action to help you physically battle with the situation in your mind, just as if it were unfolding in front of you. Your body cannot take the risk of your thoughts being 'just thoughts', as this mechanism is intended to save and preserve your life. Consider how you experience this feeling when faced with actual stress or danger and it energizes you to act quickly.

As I lay in bed that night, imagining that my husband had died, my body responded with an automatic stress response. It was as if I allowed my heart to be dragged through the heartbreak unnecessarily. When you notice your body ramping up along with your thoughts, use an interruptive technique such as counting back from 100 in threes in order to halt the rumination. Then begin to extend your exhale (for example, breathe in deeply for 4, and exhale fully for a longer count of 6 or 7). These two mechanisms help you regain control of the thinking, rational part of your brain when the emotional part is threatening to take over. It tells your body that you're safe, that the stress response is unneeded, that the story is just a story, and your sympathetic nervous response can step down.

As you manage your anxiety, you are less likely to feel that physical sense of panic. If you don't find ways to calm the whirlwind of fear that rises up in you every time you think about losing someone you love, then you will have a strong association between thinking about loss and experiencing a sense of panic. When this is the case, no wonder thinking about the inevitable truth of loss feels too painful. As you confront the essence of your anxiety, and your lack of true control over life's curve balls, you can come to terms with it.

4. Address trauma and phobia of death

Traumatic experiences and phobia of death (called thanatophobia) mean that even thinking of losing a loved one can induce a feeling of panic. Distressing flashbacks and nightmares are common symptoms of post-traumatic stress. You may also feel strong, distressing emotions arise if you encounter anything that is reminiscent of the traumatic experience you faced.

My client Fi came to see me to discuss her relationship with her mother. Her mother was traumatized after the death of her niece (Fi's cousin) in a way that her father wasn't. Her father had an established support network of friends from his college days and, as a therapist, he had tools to help him cope.

Fi's father felt able to talk to the family about his grief. He would often talk about grief with Fi and would encourage her to allow the waves of sadness to ebb and flow. Her mother internalized and sought to numb her grief through means of alcohol and overworking. It seemed to Fi that, even years later, for her mother it was as if the loss had happened only days before. Her mother would avoid music that reminded her of loss and would immediately turn off any TV show that approached themes of death as the pain sat so close to the surface.

As Fi continued to work with me, her mother had 'finally agreed to see a therapist'. Fi was overjoyed and would tell me how, as her mother sought ways to address and process her grief, it was freeing her up to enjoy life more in the present: 'There is more light in her eyes. It's like she's living in the now rather than stuck in the past.'

If this chapter has stirred up lots of uncomfortable feelings for you, please know that where there is help, there is hope. I highly recommend seeking some therapeutic support. Turn to the Helpful Contacts section at the back of the book for guidance on where you can find help. Right now, it might feel too much to even think about losing someone you love, let alone stare the uncomfortable truth in the face. But with the right support, one day you'll peek through your fingers and, in time, you'll be able to look at it for a little longer with growing acceptance and the freedom that comes with living with less fear.

5. Establish and widen your support network

You need support throughout life, regardless of the challenges you will face in your path. This isn't weakness or failure but human necessity! Conversely, many cultures encourage individualism and applaud you when you show that you are strong and self-sufficient. My client Pete encountered loss as a child after his brother passed away: 'My parents took the photos of him off the wall and we never spoke of Miles again. I wanted to, but I didn't know how to because I just worried about upsetting them.' Many once close-knit communities have evolved to be collections of houses where everything important goes on behind closed doors, and there's a fear of judgement or burdening someone if you were to share life's messiness or pain with others.

If you find it painful to consider the truth that you'll lose people because you don't know where you would turn, then establish and broaden your support network. Open up to those you know in order to deepen your friendships, or find new friends by engaging in group activities or dusting off a dormant hobby. Knowing that people are there for you will serve you well regardless of what lies ahead, as we humans are creatures of community.

Conclusion

I remember asking my mother whether she would rather not have known my little sister for the six years of her life than know her and go through the pain of losing her as she did. And her reply is something I return to when I am fearing more than accepting the truth of loss: 'I am grateful for every single day of loving her.' Yes, love and loss go hand in hand, such is the truth of life. But many will tell you that: 'Love? It is worth it all.'

Imagine a big gold coin sitting in the palm of your hand. On one side the word *love* is engraved. Think about the love you give and have in your life. The more love, the bigger the coin. Now, turn the coin over. You see the word *vulnerability*. This is the risk of loss and heartache, because the more you love, the more you have to lose. Oh, I wish it were not true, but we simply cannot have one without the other. In truth, your life is made rich with the love that you have within it.

So, continue to seek an acceptance of the truth that you will lose people you love and let it motivate you to live and love more intentionally.

JOURNAL POINTS

1. What feeds your own fear of losing someone?

2. Which words did you find most comforting in this chapter? Write them down and reflect on them further by adding your own thoughts.

3. Would you benefit from therapeutic support for traumatic grief or fear of loss? Make a pledge to seek support by writing what step you will take.

To love is worth the loss

10.

I am Going to Die

Diving headfirst into the uncomfortable truth

Well, we're finishing off with a bang here, aren't we? I'm going to take it gently, I promise. I know this big truth is one that we'll all be challenged to confront at some point, yet it can be life-changing to move further into an acceptance that your life won't last forever.

How old you are and what you've been through in life will impact on how you read this chapter. Perhaps you feel like you have your whole life ahead of you, and you don't yet have any wrinkles to tell you otherwise. Maybe you're arriving at this chapter having nursed a parent at the end of their life or maybe the aftershocks of traumatic loss are still rippling through your days. Whether you have spent time writing a will or want to shut family members down

275

when they bring up the topic of death, you're not alone. There will be words in this chapter to soothe, encourage and inspire you towards acceptance.

Regardless of how many tricks and hacks we reach out for to prevent the slow and consistent decline of our bodies, although we can sometimes improve our health we can never evade our eventual death. As Irvin Yalom says in his book *Staring at the Sun: Overcoming the Terror of Death*, 'The more unlived your life, the greater your death anxiety. The more you fail to experience your life fully, the more you will fear death.' As I have found ways to live more fully, I am a little less fearful of my own ending. But in the same way, as I have found ways to become more accepting of my own death, I have also begun to feel like I'm living more fully. So, let's step into this topic together, with the hope that finding gentle acceptance will also find you enjoying a much more 'lived' life.

Sometimes I stand outside or lie on the cold grass and stare at the stars. I make myself dizzy thinking about how long those stars have been in existence and how many generations before me have gazed up at them too. There is something powerful in recognizing the vast picture of life: that we exist in an era between those past and those to come, in times which we won't be here to experience for ourselves. In those moments I am held between awe and wonder and the humility of feeling acutely small. Life feels so long in some ways, especially as I get caught up in the stresses, large and small, of daily life. In other ways I feel like I have whiplash from the speed of life. How am I thirty-eight, with a mortgage, three children, a cat and almost fifteen years of marriage? How am I a fully fledged grown-up when it feels like moments ago I was a child playing in the woodland, scrapping with my younger brother over how best to build a den?

How do we find meaning in our existence when it's both long and challenging, yet at the same time seemingly over in a heartbeat? How do we ground ourselves when the little things in our life feel so huge, but we are so small in the context of a limitless universe?

The fear of death is the biggest source of human anxiety and regret. I have worked with hundreds of clients over the years and we've always, in some context, touched on awareness of life's speed, fragility and meaning. Some clients feel empowered to make more conscious decisions when considering their own limited life, whereas others find their anxiety fuelled by this same awareness. When we think about death, we are confronted with the truth of our powerlessness and fragility as humans. We can plan and attempt to control every aspect of our lives, but ultimately our life could end at any given moment. It is so humbling, isn't it? I'm not wishing to draw you into an existential crisis, though, fear not. I am going to help you use this uncomfortable truth to empower you to live more intentionally rather than more fearfully.

We have vastly different experiences and emotions surrounding the awareness of our own death, from point-blank denial at one end to a constant, underlying preoccupation and fear of it at the other. In an ideal, perfect world, death would only happen in old age. My mother has worked as a physiotherapist in a children's hospice and as a volunteer counsellor in an adult one. She recalls how it's not uncommon an experience for staff to see people smile or even say someone's name as they die, as if they have been reunited with a loved one.

When you're young, thinking about your own death can feel like a terrifying prospect. Perhaps you've not lost anyone or experienced healthy grief. It can be hard to imagine that as people move through life, they may well have a more relaxed approach to their death as they age, even feeling comfortable to reflect on it or to focus on the logistics of 'tying life up' before they leave, sorting through attics and getting paperwork in order to relieve stress from friends and family. In ageing or sickness, death may even be welcomed, accepted or deemed a relief.

My client Graham sighed as he eased himself into the armchair in our therapy session. He had been told that the cancer which had sat dormant for the last ten years had spread and was now untreatable. 'I'd become complacent,' he told me. 'The cancer scared me at first, but with treatment it just existed, in my body, doing nothing. I accepted it and got on with life.

'Only when the doctor sat there and told me the results of some recent tests did I really get that feeling people talk about where "life flashes before your eyes". In some ways, he gave me a death sentence. But it really feels like a life sentence. I've never felt so alive. I've never loved so hard, appreciated so much or been so calm and careless of the things that truly don't matter. I feel like I'm living for the first time, truly. I wish I could share some of this feeling with others, bottle it if you will, so that everyone could really live while they can. I see friends sleepwalk through life, rolling from one life milestone to the next.'

It was true, Graham's body was increasingly frail with each session, but his eyes were full of life. In a following session he told me excitedly how he'd learned on social media about the idea of a 'living funeral' and had been inspired to plan his own funeral while he was still alive in order to be able to get everyone together. 'Don't get me wrong,' he said, 'I have my dark moments and I am in pain. I am a bit scared about what it feels like to die, but I don't have long to live and I want to really live it.'

I hope that we can be moved by Graham's story. I don't want to wait until near death to truly live. In this chapter, I hope that you'll feel empowered, because when we accept death as the backdrop to life, we are faced with the incredible choice to live more intentionally and to value the preciousness within it.

My story

I used to be very fearful thinking about death; it was a topic I'd try to avoid talking about. I have avoided attending funerals over the years because it just felt too painful and would prompt feelings of my own grief over the loss of my sister that I had pushed down deep within me. The more I've processed my grief through therapy, just letting the feelings arise and abate, the more open I've become to thinking about life against the backdrop of death.

I went for a walk with a friend during the pandemic. We'd been musing about the passing of time and living purposefully. Trust me, I don't always have such philosophical conversations with friends, but with this one I do and I love it. We can move from discussing our favourite box set to the meaning of life in a matter of minutes.

'I sometimes imagine that I'm standing in a queue along with every other person in the world. When you get to the front, you die,' she said. 'I don't know what number I am in the queue, whether I'm near the front or part way down, but I'm in it and every second I'm moving closer to the front, closer to my death.' What struck me was that she said this with total acceptance, not fear. Had she not said it in such a matter-of-fact way, I might have thought, 'Well, that's absolutely horrifying.' I was intrigued by the blasé way she said it. She had lost her mother as a teenager; I had lost my sister as a child. We had both lost people close to us out of the normal order of things and yet she viewed her own death in a different way to me.

I decided to continue contemplating this queue metaphor. It jarred at first; it felt uncomfortable to think about something I'd spent so long avoiding. I began to repeat 'I am going to die' to myself. Perhaps the conversation I had with her was unconsciously the conception of this book.

I hold my own death a lot more in mind these days and I have a deep recognition of the passing of time. Maybe it's because I don't feel so young any more. I'm watching my children grow and my parents age. As I lie down in bed, I'm aware that another day has passed, and as I wake, I feel an increasing reverence for the gift of another. Even if the day ahead is tough, I am grateful to be alive because I don't assume that I always will be. This increasing awareness of the passing of time, and all that it means about my own inevitable death, is helping me to live more intentionally.

If my life is going to end, I want to live it as well as I can. If I don't know when that's going to happen, then I want to make sure I grasp it with both hands. I want to make decisions that align with my passions; I want to find meaning; I want to spend time with those I love. I want to try to make sure I'm not wasting my days and my attention. I dance constantly between getting caught up in the thick of life and zooming out to welcome the perspective that acceptance of its ending brings.

Another thing that personally grounds me as I reflect on the meaning of life and the purpose of my existence is spiritual practice. I have a deep belief in a higher power which provides me with a sense of understanding as to my important place in the lineage of my life and the generations that have come before me and will come after.

My life may be a link in a long chain, but the work I do on myself and for others has the power to strengthen that chain and benefit those who live beyond me. Over the last six months I have been waking early to engage in spiritual reflection which has given me a greater sense of meaning, self-worth and purpose. So while existential philosopher Nietzsche suggested that life is inherently meaningless, in the vein of existential therapy, I would personally suggest that life is 'anchorless' until you find the things that give you a solid sense of meaning.

I have stopped getting quite so frustrated with myself or going to bed with regret for all the moments that I didn't make the most of, the opportunities I didn't take, the hours that passed in a blur, the parenting guilt. I try to live intentionally when I remember to, and whenever I have decisions to make around work or relationships I try to take into account the bigger picture of life and it's fleetingness.

Why deny?

Here are some reasons you might feel more fearful than accepting when it comes to the uncomfortable truth of the inevitability of your death.

- **Because you're not happy with the trajectory of your life** If you're not happy with where you're at in life then it can be hard to think about the fact that you have limited time on this earth. You may have set yourself particular goals or 'should's for certain ages, such as 'I should have found a partner by the age of thirty-five' or 'I should have found a job I'm happy in by twenty-five'. When you place a framework on your life, or you don't find enough of a sense of meaning and purpose at the stage you're currently at, you can feel a pressure or a rush if you haven't hit your goals in time.

- **You don't know who to talk to about death** If your family or wider culture avoid talking about death then it can feel like a taboo topic. You may not feel comfortable to talk openly about it, or to bring it up as something to muse or contemplate on, because you can see the discomfort of others when you do so. Maybe your family didn't openly express or welcome feelings of grief or sadness, so it feels tough to talk about topics that can stir up these feelings in yourself and others. Perhaps you lost someone traumatically or experienced a situation in which you were faced with near death and find it a very powerful, emotionally loaded topic to contemplate.

- **Concern about how you're going to die** This is totally understandable, right? There is so much about life which is unknown, yet the one certainty is that it ends for everybody at some point. You may have witnessed someone dying peacefully, or you may have seen or heard of traumatic, sudden deaths, people who died before their time, leaving a trail of heartbreak. One reason to avoid living with the acceptance of death is fear of how it will happen.

Which of these reasons feels most pertinent for you? Understanding why we find certain uncomfortable truths harder to face than others can be helpful as we may need to address things that really stand in the way of moving forward. Perhaps you'd benefit from some therapeutic support to help process a traumatic loss. It might be that the realization that you're not where you had hoped you would be at this point in your life prompts you to mix things up a bit or to be more intentional in certain areas of your life.

The benefits of embracing this uncomfortable truth

The more you become aware of the benefits of beginning to embrace the vastly uncomfortable truth that your life is finite, the more you will want to enjoy living more intentionally. My hope is that as you read through these benefits, you'll start to recognize quite how freeing it could be to live life against the backdrop of death in the realization that each day is a gift, not a given.

- **You stop sweating the small stuff** The more you accept that your life is limited, the more grateful you will feel for each day and good thing within it, and the more able to recognize the privileges and beauty in your life. It's all too easy to get bogged down in the detail, or find yourself making decisions that don't really align with your values because 'there's plenty of time for that'. I once sat in the hospital, waiting for a scan, beside an elderly lady. As she began to have a coughing fit, I offered her a cup of water from the machine next to me. We got chatting. She told me she had terminal lung cancer and urged me to make the most of the life I had. 'Don't sweat the small stuff,' she said as she held my gaze with tears in her eyes. I don't want to wait until the end of my life to have this valuable perspective. While I cannot always drink up every moment, as we identified in Chapter 4, I can choose to look through this lens whenever I remember to.

- **You stop putting life on hold** Can you remember the 'when, then' game from Chapter 4? 'When I have the job I want, I'll be happy. When it gets to the weekend, I'll rest. When I've worked on my confidence, I'll share more of my opinion. When my parents get old, then I'll start seeing them more.' As you embrace the truth that you'll die one day, you'll stop holding off from choosing to live a full and authentic life for another day or another year, and you'll start living more while you certainly can.

- **You prioritize important relationships** One of the dying's biggest regrets is that they didn't spend enough time with those they loved most. When you choose to live with an accepting awareness of your own death, then you are more likely to benefit from the perspective it brings on what is important to you in how you spend your time and resources. You may be more intentional about who you spend your time with and which relationships you invest your precious energy in, meaning you'll enjoy more richness of connection in your life.

- **You're more mentally and logistically prepared for death** The less you contemplate and feel accepting of death as the conclusion of life, the more you'll feel sideswept when you hear of death and dying. For the older generations, avoiding thinking about death means that you are unprepared: maybe wills aren't updated and important paperwork has been lost. A family friend of mine, on being diagnosed with terminal cancer, wrote a series of letters for her children to read on every birthday until they hit eighteen. Her acceptance of her own death meant that she was able to think beyond it, as painful and grief-filled as that must have been for her. When we choose to move out of a place of denial, we recognize what choices we may have in how we approach our own death, and what legacy we wish to leave behind.

You may well be able to add further thoughts to this list. I encourage you to think about the impact that avoiding this uncomfortable truth might have for you. Consider if you were to die in five years – how would that shift your perspective on how you spend your days, who you see, which relationships you invest in? Some people find it immensely powerful to imagine their own funerals in order to engage in considering their death as a prompt to live more intentionally. It is becoming increasingly popular to enact death through meditation. In Seoul, South Korea, a 'Death Experience School' run by a funeral home even gives people the chance to lie in coffins, compose a farewell letter and have a funeral portrait taken.

Five ways to live with the truth that you will die

How, then, when contemplating your own death as a way of living life more fully, do you move from fear to acceptance? Here are five tips that have been so helpful for me.

1. Allow yourself to dance in and out of awareness

Accepting the uncomfortable truth of your own death is absolutely to be viewed as a process. One which you'll likely never feel truly comfortable with or deeply accepting of. Don't pressure yourself to ever feel completely at ease with it, that isn't the aim here. The aim is not to live fully in fear of your life coming to a conclusion but instead to find gentle acceptance that leads you to live more authentically and intentionally.

There will be times in life when the daily demands are so absorbing that you are just embedded in the everyday. There will also be times of challenge, loss and those moments where 'normal' hangs in the balance when you may find your attention fully drawn to the fragility of life.

My client Stan, on losing his partner, found himself in a 'tug of war between being aware of the precious gift that is today, while also finding myself frustrated at the nuances of work stresses'. As he navigated grief, he became acutely conscious of how he was experiencing elements of life that his partner had learned to value: 'I was so aware of the beauty of rain upon my face, as when he was sick, John would say how it was wild he'd soon never feel it again.' Stan would pledge to make the most of his days and opportunities yet would berate himself for getting stressed over work and the 'small stuff'. We talked about how awareness of death helps us live more fully, but how being permanently fixated on the inevitability of death would prevent us from engaging in and being humanly impacted by our day-to-day life.

I sometimes think of my awareness of death as similar to looking at the sun, its blazing light so blinding it cannot be looked at for more than a moment. Other times the sun is softened and welcomes your gaze as a stunning, life-affirming sunset of pinks and oranges.

Perhaps we are forever in a grieving process for life itself. As you become aware of your mortality you are aware of that which you may one day lose. Sometimes, if I wake at night in the darkness, I feel a stark, contemplative awareness of the passing of time. I experience a pang of sadness for the day which I will not get back and a swell of excitement that I get to live another day with those I love. If I didn't allow myself to feel the loss of what has passed, I wouldn't feel the gratitude for what is still present quite as keenly.

Loss changes us. Think of how when you lose someone or something precious to you, you gain fresh appreciation for that which you still have. And in the same way as you recognize the truth of loss in your life's journey, you can touch on the same gratitude for the life you still have to live.

If you have a moment to journal, take some time to consider your feelings and fears about your own mortality. Write down some of the circumstances, decisions or relationships in your life that you might engage with differently if you were to have more acceptance of this uncomfortable truth. Choose to be open in allowing yourself to contemplate, observe and listen to others when it comes to talking about death and dying. We often fear most that which is least familiar to us, so as you discuss, debate and explore the topic with others, you may find the fear slowly ebbs away.

2. Find your meaning

Why am I here? What is the meaning of life? These questions have engaged discussion throughout history. Humans need to experience a sense of significance, a belief that we matter somehow, to ourselves and others, and that we play a meaningful part in the wider community. To live with an inherent sense of inner worth allows you to cease spending your life searching for validation through achievement, opinion and possessions, but to fully engage feeling safe and secure.

My client Miranda had an experience one morning that led her to find a whole new level of meaning to her life: 'I headed into work extra early one morning because of an impending deadline. A soup van was delivering breakfast to the homeless who'd sleep around the Tube station. I'd never seen it before. I kept thinking about it all day, recalling how people had handed out steaming pots of porridge to those who'd been sleeping on the freezing city floor.' This sparked something off in her. 'I lay in bed thinking of those sleeping outside and the next day I searched online to find the charity who'd been handing out food.'

A few weeks later, Miranda caught an early train into the city to join those handing out porridge for an hour before she headed into the office. She met a whole new community of people who were passionate about using some of their available resources to help others. 'Something about it shocked me out of my almost hypnotic state of getting up, working, working out and going to bed. Handing out porridge once a week woke me up to life where I'd been on autopilot. I felt a sense of purpose and meaning that I hadn't fully experienced before. I'd tried to find it in work, but it hadn't hit the spot like this did.' Within months, Miranda had gathered a few colleagues together who were increasingly keen to find other ways to support those sleeping on the streets.

To discover your own sense of meaning, ask yourself these questions: What motivates you? What would matter most if everything were to be stripped away tomorrow? How much are your decisions, your resources and the way you spend your time in line with those things? What do you live for that feeds, calms and drives you to good things and places? Or do your priorities fuel fear-based behaviour like perfectionism, people-pleasing or self-abandonment?

What excites you and when do you feel at your most peaceful, passionate, content or alive? Are you engaging in enough of these activities in your life? Take some time to write down your own manifesto. Include your values, whatever they may be. Consider how they shape your priorities, goals and decisions. Discovering a sense of purpose prompts feelings of enthusiasm and accomplishment as you live in alignment with your values.

Engaging in spirituality further offers people a sense of meaning. How much thought do you give to what happens beyond life? Millions all over the world explore the meaning of life and death through spirituality as it invites us to reach out for something bigger than ourselves, offering a framework for life and beyond.

Some people find that involvement in a faith community gives them a sense of belonging, strength, purpose, confidence and comfort. Others may find meaning through nature, other human beings or, like me, through a higher power or personal God. Your spirituality may change and evolve through your life experiences. What gives you comfort in some circumstances may do so less in others, so that you continue to reach and search for something more.

My personal spiritual quest has led me to embrace a sense of purpose for my own life and a firm belief that I will be reunited with my loved ones when I die; that a part of me will continue beyond death, so while death is final in the flesh, I have a spiritual soul that will live on. You may dispute that with me or you may find comfort in that same thought for yourself. Some believe that you return to live in another form dependent on how well you have lived. For those who embrace a belief in an afterlife, it can help cultivate acceptance when it comes to being aware that you will die.

Another way to explore your meaning is to recognize your successes. Look back over your life and allow yourself to be proud of your achievements and the relationships you've formed. You have positively impacted people's lives along the way and that is something to draw a sense of meaning from. Kindness, friendship and contributing to community are all ways to cultivate a meaningful life. The more you lean into your own sense of meaning and purpose, the less you will look to the world and those around you for validation of your existence.

So, question your meaning and purpose and get new clarity on what your values are, so that as decisions arise you can ensure you are living and acting in line with these things. As you live a meaningful, relational, wholehearted life, it becomes a strong foundation from which to reflect on your own meaning and mortality.

3. Make decisions against the backdrop of death

When decisions arise, recall the truth that you will one day die. Let it bring clarity and direction in a positive way. This isn't about anxiety and fear but about welcoming the truth in order to challenge whether you're acting authentically and in line with your values or not.

I remember feeling really preoccupied with a housemate at university who struggled to have healthy friendships. While it was obvious the issue was reflected in all of her friendships, of course, I took it very personally and felt desperate to make it right. On expressing this to another friend, she said, 'Anna, you won't know her in five years.' I hadn't really thought about projecting into the future as a way of challenging what I felt was important in the present. But it really helped and I began to use that concept quite a lot.

In one of our sessions, my client Saz found this concept really useful when dealing with stresses around her lease ending on her flat. 'I was filled with stress at trying to find a new place and trying to line up the timings with having to move out of my old flat. Thinking about how in five years' time I'd be safely living in a flat somewhere felt really reassuring. The details were all up in the air and needed my time and attention, but in truth, in the grand scheme of things, I knew I'd be okay.'

As a way of acting upon this, consider your current worries and concerns and ask yourself, 'Do I need to be worrying about this so much when next week it will be just a memory?' Maybe you do need to spend time considering how to act or react. Perhaps this concern is worthy of your headspace and energy. Or perhaps you recognize through the lens of this question that you need to choose to untether a particular thought, like cutting the ropes which tether a hot air balloon, releasing it from your mind.

I guess becoming more accepting and less fearful of the uncomfortable truth that you'll die is a little like this. It helps you consider what is important to you and challenges where you're placing your time and energy.

Maybe we witness less death in our current culture. Historically, families didn't move so far apart from one another. Generations stayed within a town or county. Unlike the present day, when families are often spread across different geographical locations due to moving for work and study, your lives would have intermingled far more than they do now. You'd have been a significant part of each other's community and support network. I don't see many old people in my life these days. I live on a development populated by young families. My friends and direct community are also men and women in their thirties and forties. In my day-to-day life, I don't draw from the wisdom of the older generations, nor do I see many old people navigating their final years. The more we are drawn to people like ourselves, the less we benefit from the input of those who truly are older and wiser. But, importantly, when it comes to accepting the uncomfortable truth of death, the less we are engaging with those who are nearing the end of their lives, the less likely we are to engage in our own lives, holding death in awareness.

A few years ago, there were some beautiful photographs on social media of old people holding signs portraying their wisdom and advice to younger generations: *Be kind to everyone, Make time for those you love, Let go of the small grievances.* In situations where you live alongside the new and the old, and it's normal to see people at both the beginning and end of their life, then perhaps it's easier to think about life against the backdrop of death. But if you don't have that now, then cultivate it by bringing it to your awareness. It will feel more natural in time, I promise.

4. Learn how to grieve well

Learning how to acknowledge the small griefs and losses of life, in time, helps you to become more accepting of the big ones. When you feel sadness at a season of life ending, or you've lost something precious or important to you, just allow yourself to feel how you do without judgement. Grieve the loss of treasured items, pets, jobs, dreams and loved ones, and don't rush it, or put rules around how long you should feel sad, or how sad you should feel.

Dotted all over the world, you'll find Death Cafes. They are organized gatherings where people freely talk about death, which just shows how it's something that's little discussed and yet such discussion is deeply desired by so many people in societies everywhere. If you want to talk more about death, find those who are open to doing so. Talking about death helps us untangle our feelings about it and chips away at the taboo.

If, like me, you've been through a traumatic loss that fuels fear of death, then seek therapeutic support. When you bury something inside of yourself, it doesn't disappear, it just waits for an opportunity to surface and be validated. Perhaps historic, unprocessed feelings of grief and loss reappear or feel reinvigorated when you face a present loss. My client Sam came to speak with me to explore why losing his cat felt so painful. 'I couldn't work, focus or cope with day-to-day life,' he said. 'I kept thinking, "What is wrong with me? It's sad, but it's my cat, not my child or my partner."' He felt fearful that he wouldn't be able to live through the loss of a person, as he felt utterly devastated by the loss of his pet. We were able to determine that the grief he hadn't felt able to understand or express as an eight-year-old, when he lost his grandfather, was resurfacing.

Just as with trauma, loss can trigger other experiences and memories of loss, and this can be more pronounced when grief has been inhibited in some way. For Sam, his mother was so pained by the loss of her father (his grandfather), that she wasn't able to help him understand or navigate his own feelings. In our sessions, we made space for Sam to speak about and grieve both the loss of his grandfather and his cat. He found this immensely useful and, with time, the overwhelming sense of sadness he'd experienced softened to make day-to-day life feel more manageable.

How do you grieve? There is no one-size-fits-all rule, timeline or road map, as much as we love to know whether we're doing something 'right'. I recommend simply acknowledging the emotions that you feel, without judgement or 'rules' such as 'I should feel happier now' or 'I shouldn't be feeling joyful today'. Know that how you feel will be unique to you and your emotions may be triggered unexpectedly. Express your feelings through talking, writing or finding a creative outlet – just let them out. Let others know what you do and don't need from them, and be prepared for these things to shift and change as the days, months and years go by.

So, grieve the losses, both big and small, and choose not to shy away from talking about death to those who are up for chatting. As you honour your own emotions, you will be able to better experience life's sadnesses, but you'll more openly welcome the rich joys too.

5. Welcoming new beginnings and good times

It is true that everything ends. But think about the seasons and cycles of nature. The daytime moves into darkness, but the light brings with it a brand-new day. Rain makes way for sunshine and winter recedes with the first shoots of spring. Nothing stays the same for long. Draw on this promise through life, through tough times and heartache. As you choose to become more accepting of life's losses and the closing of seasons, you are invited to appreciate the shoots of life and the diamonds that glisten in the rubble there to be found.

'My relationship ended last year,' shared my client Antonio. 'At first, I was so angry because I felt like I'd wasted years of my life trying to make something work that didn't. I thought we were in it for the long haul.' As we talked through the intricacies of the relationship ending, Antonio felt more able to reflect on that period of his life as a 'mixed bag' rather than just a waste: 'I saw how I had learned important stuff about how to nurture (and how not to nurture!) relationships that I will take on into the rest of my life. I had grown in some ways through those years and have also learned so much about myself through the break-up, strengthening some of my relationships through needing some support.'

Things can be tough, but not everything is. Life can be sad, but not everything is. Validate your emotions as they arise and choose also to bring balance by seeking the privileges and light within the season of life that you're in.

Another way to welcome new beginnings and to help accept your finite life is to reject the cultural narrative that as you move through life you become somehow lesser. Our culture worships youth and perfection but in truth, while each season and stage of life comes with a loss of sorts, there is new life and growth to find too.

Many people discover as they mature that people-pleasing loses its grip, perfectionism loses its allure and there is freedom in finding more confidence in your authenticity. Choosing to accept the truth of your ageing and death means that you can be intentional about addressing anything that robs you of being your authentic self rather than waiting for age to bring the wisdom. I don't want to wait until I'm seventy to worry less about what people think of me, because who says I'll make it to seventy? I want to live a full life now.

Being more aware of your own mortality does not need to be doom and gloom at all! If your focus is on what you could lose rather than on what you have, then anxiety is likely to be playing a part. Anxiety impacts your ability to see and engage in the goodness in front of you. Consider a time when you have been doing something you really enjoy, but your mind has been elsewhere. Perhaps you have been worried about something going wrong, or fixated on the clock as you have somewhere to be afterwards. Think about how your ability to enjoy that experience was restricted because of your worry or concern. If you're rushing through a walk, you're far less likely to enjoy a beautiful view or have the chance to marvel at the flowers in your path. In the same way, fear of your life ending prevents you from absorbing some of the goodness that is there within it.

Anxiety is often focused on the potential loss of safety or 'life as you know it'. The antidote to this anxiety is to draw your awareness to the good things that are happening in your life now. So, when it comes to thinking about your mortality, bring balance to any fear by choosing also to focus on the wonder within it. As you become aware of your white-knuckle-hug moments, you have the choice to ease your grip, lean into gratitude and inhale the presence of the person in your company.

And for those times when the pain of the moment is raw and overwhelming, know that this too will soften and pass, just as the depth of winter gives way to spring.

Conclusion

In this final chapter, you've gazed right into the uncomfortable truth of your own limited life. I hope I have helped open your eyes to how living in denial or fear of this truth challenges your ability to live a full and wholehearted life. It doesn't mean you need to live as if you'll die tomorrow, because imagine the decisions we'd make if that were to be true!

By living against the backdrop of your death, you'll find yourself making more intentional decisions and inhaling life's good stuff more consciously. Let the awareness be like the newly hung wallpaper on your living-room wall. At first you notice it all the time, your eyes move straight to the pattern that wasn't there before. But as the days go by, you feel less surprised by it. Your mind has just accepted it as part of the room. Go gently on yourself as you dance back and forth between awareness and denial, and remember that it is meant to be this way.

JOURNAL POINTS

1. How does it feel to think about the uncomfortable truth of your death?

2. What is the main reason you have tried to avoid thinking about this truth?

3. Take some time to write down thoughts about where you find meaning.

———

Accepting that I will die one day can prompt me to live more fully in the present

My Final Letter to You

Dear Reader,

Thank you for trusting me to tackle these huge truths with you. A few years ago some of them would have felt unbearable for me to spend longer than a few moments considering them, and perhaps at points it felt really confronting for you too. I promise you that as you keep reflecting on them, your fear and anxiety will soften as you begin to accept them and make decisions in light of them.

Keep coming back to this book, to the truths that you need to face, so that you can become a little more unstuck in areas that hold you back. For example, if you're struggling with people-pleasing, spend some time rereading Chapter 1. If you've heard some sad news and are faced with your fear of something bad happening, seek some words from Chapter 8 to encourage and calm you.

You get to do this thing called 'life' once. And you deserve to live it to the fullest you possibly can without being tethered by fear and anxiety. Our culture will sell you the narrative that gaining more mastery over your life is the key to living with less fear and anxiety. If you can predict bad things happening, if you can access all the knowledge in the world, if you can get all the answers, then you will fear less. But, in truth, we have never felt more powerless, disconnected, anxious and fearful.

This book is your invitation to try a different way. Instead of seeking more mastery over your life, instead of trying to find more ways to control, I invite you to lean into the truth of your powerlessness, your limits, your vulnerability and your lack of control. When you truly know what you're working with, you can live more intentionally.

When you are aware that some people won't like you, you can preserve energy from trying to change the minds of those who need to misunderstand you. When you accept that bad things will happen, you can stop bracing yourself through the good times. When you accept that you will one day die, you can choose to seek the things that bring you joy and meaning, rather than hold off for another day or decade. The more you come to terms with the limits of your resources, the more you can allow others to step in and fill the gaps with their strengths.

If you tend towards perfectionism, choose not to apply perfectionism to this journey you're on. I have a little saying I repeat to myself: 'More of the time, not all of the time.' Learning to accept the uncomfortable truths is a bumpy upwards graph rather than a neat, slick trajectory. We all want to hide from these truths sometimes – that's not cowardice, that's human. Irvin Yalom muses that to live with a constant awareness of death is like trying to stare the sun in the face: 'You can only stand so much of it.'

So, give yourself permission to dance in and out of awareness of the uncomfortable truths of life. And when you do glance straight in the face of an uncomfortable truth, allow it to enable you to live more fully and intentionally where you can. I urge you to have a huge amount of grace and patience for yourself as you dance between acceptance and denial. Just keep dancing, all the same. Keep dancing and keep living, truly living.

In time you will come to realize just how beautiful, freeing and life-giving it can be to face these ten uncomfortable truths.

With love, Anna xx

Helpful Contacts

CALM – Campaign Against Living Miserably
https://www.thecalmzone.net
A helpline for those in the UK who are feeling down for any reason.

Cruse
https://www.cruse.org.uk
Bereavement support charity, offering free support to those who have lost a loved one.

Depression UK
http://depressionuk.org
A national self-help organization helping people cope with depression.

Help Guide
https://www.helpguide.org
Helping people make changes to help their mental health.

The Hub of Hope

https://hubofhope.co.uk

Enter your postcode to find local support networks and charities.

Mind

https://www.mind.org.uk

Providing advice and support to empower anyone experiencing a mental health challenge.

The Samaritans

https://www.samaritans.org

Volunteers available to listen every moment of every day.

You can also call 116123 and speak to a trained volunteer day or night.

Author's Note

I wrote this book in two weeks. I typed fervently between meetings on work days, before the kids woke for breakfast and in snatched moments before I flopped on to the sofa with dinner in the evening. I took a risk and wrote it before any publisher agreed to print it – actually before any publisher even knew how the idea had been impatiently sitting in my mind like an overdue bill on the kitchen counter that needs to be settled. I told my wonderful literary agent that I was just going to write regardless of what happened next.

My fourth book hadn't hit the shelves yet. It was an utter relief to pour my thoughts into my keyboard and see this book come to be. I was so happy in those two weeks, in my creative flow. I'd conclude each chapter and send it to a handful of friends, eagerly awaiting their feedback.

I have never had such a starkly clear idea about a book. It came to me like a vision, complete with the title and even the colour of the cover. I tapped the title, the cover design and the whole format along with each of the ten truths into my iPhone as I stood next to my bed in a hotel in Warwick, about to give a TEDx talk on motherhood guilt.

Days after typing the final sentences of the first draft, one of those ground-shaking, heartbeat-pausing curve balls hit our lives. As I returned to edit it months later, I was enthralled by how true the words had been for me, that to live in this way meant to live more fully, both through the skyscraper highs and valley lows.

The key to surviving hadn't been to guard myself against potential pain through controlling everything around me but to lean into vulnerability and rely on the strength of others. Instead of shaking my fist at life's unfairness, I was able to channel that same energy into self-compassion and seeking habits that would support me through the storm.

Before I wrote this book, the different approaches to anxiety were already changing my life. But through the following months, they were put to the test. I recognized how an increasing acceptance of these uncomfortable truths forms a steadfast anchor to keep us secure, not only in the day-to-day mundane but also through times when life's tidal waves hit. Sure, our boat shakes in the roaring waves, but underneath the thrashing current, the anchor holds.

So, I hope this book speaks to you deeply. I hope it gently shakes you free of living fearfully and nudges you towards a fuller, more authentic existence as you so deserve.

I hope that you will join me in sticking a flag into the ground and proclaiming:

'I refuse to spend my whole life living a half-life.'

Bibliography

Camus, Albert, *Notebooks: 1935–1951*, trans. by Philip Malcolm Waller Thody and J. O'Brien, new edition (Boston, MA: Marlowe & Co., 1998).

Carlson, Richard, *Don't Sweat the Small Stuff: Simple Ways to Keep the Little Things from Overtaking Your Life* (London: Hodder & Stoughton, 1998).

Frankl, Viktor E., *Man's Search for Meaning* (1946) (London: Rider Classics, 2021).

Hoffman, Louis, 'A Cultural Crisis of Responsibility: Responding to a Denial of Our Humanity', New Existentialists Posts, Saybrook University, 6 May 2014, https://www.saybrook.edu/2014/05/06/05-06-14

Hubbard, Elbert, *Little Journeys to the Homes of American Statesmen* (New York, NY: G. P. Putnam's Sons, 1898).

BIBLIOGRAPHY

Jung, Carl, *Complex Archetype Symbol in the Psychology of C. G. Jung*, ed. by Jolande Jacobi, trans. from German by Ralph Manheim (Abingdon: Routledge, 1999).

Levy, Marc, *If Only It Were True*, republished as *Just Like Heaven* (London: HarperCollins, 2005).

Murakami, Haruki, *South of the Border, West of the Sun* (Tokyo: Kodansha, 1992); English trans. by Philip Gabriel (London: Vintage, 2000).

Nietzsche, Friedrich, *The Gay Science* (1882) (Edinburgh: Edinburgh University Press, 2021).

Smail, David, *Illusion and Reality: The Meaning of Anxiety* (London: J. M. Dent, 1984).

Yalom, Irvin D., *Existential Psychotherapy* (New York, NY: Basic Books, 1980); *When Nietzsche Wept* (New York, NY: Basic Books, 1992); *Staring at the Sun: Overcoming the Terror of Death* (Hoboken, NJ: Jossey-Bass, 2008); *A Matter of Death and Life* (Stanford, CA: Redwood Press, 2021).